MEDICINE AND JEWISH LAW

Volume I

edited by
FRED ROSNER, M.D.

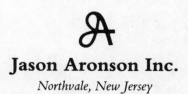

Jason Aronson Inc.
Northvale, New Jersey
London

First Softcover Edition—1993

This book was set in 11 pt. Bem by Lind Graphics of Upper Saddle River, New Jersey, and printed by Haddon Craftsmen in Scranton, Pennsylvania.

Library of Congress Cataloging-in-Publication Data

(Revised for vol. 2)

Medicine and Jewish law.

   "The Raphael [i.e. Rephael] Society, Health Care
Section of the Association of Orthodox Jewish
Scientists (AOJS), sponsored an International
Physicians' Conference on Medicine and Halachah
(Jewish law), which was held at the Fifth Avenue
Synagogue in New York City on January 1–2, 1989 . . .
The content of these proceedings is the basis of this
book"—Foreword, v. 1.
   Includes bibliographical references and index.
   1. Medicine—Religious aspects—Judaism. 2. Medical
ethics. 2. Ethics, Jewish. 3. Medical laws and
legislation (Jewish law). I. Rosner, Fred.
II. Association of Orthodox Jewish Scientists. Rephael
Society, Health Care Section. III. International
Physicians' Conference on Medicine and Halachah
(1st : 1989 : New York, N.Y.).
BM538.H43M43 1990   296.3'85642   89-49410
ISBN 0-87668-790-7 (vol. 1, hb)
ISBN 1-56821-028-0 (vol. 1, pb)
ISBN 0-87668-574-2 (vol. 2, pb)
ISBN 0-87668-681-1 (series)

Manufactured in the United States of America. Jason Aronson Inc. offers books and cassettes. For information and catalog write to Jason Aronson Inc., 230 Livingston Street, Northvale, New Jersey 07647.

This book is dedicated to the past Presidents of the Association of Orthodox Jewish Scientists, who, by virtue of their professional training, interests, activities, and hard work on behalf of AOJS, have improved the Torah way of life for Orthodox Jewish scientists throughout the modern world.

1948–1959	Eli Levine, Ph.D.
1960–1962	Elmer Offenbacher, Ph.D.
1963	Herbert Goldstein, Ph.D.
1964–1965	Azriel Rosenfeld, Ph.D.
1966–1967	Seymour Glick, M.D.
1968–1969	Leo Levi, Ph.D.
1970	Theodore Fink, Ph.D.
1971–1972	Rabbi Moshe D. Tendler, Ph.D.
1973–1974	Rabbi Paul Kahn, Ph.D.
1975–1977	Nora Smith, M.D.
1977–1978	Herbert Goldstein, Ph.D.
1979–1980	Reuben Rudman, Ph.D.
1981–1982	Lester Kaufman, A.C.S.W.
1983–1984	Erwin Friedman, Ph.D.
1985–1986	Sheldon Kornbluth, P.E.
1987–1988	Allen J. Bennett, M.D.
1989–1990	Seymour Applebaum, M.D.

CONTENTS

CONTRIBUTORS

Abraham S. Abraham, M.D.

Director, Department of Medicine, Shaare Zedek Medical Center, Jerusalem; Associate Professor of Medicine, Hebrew University

Allen J. Bennett, M.D.

Private practice of internal medicine, New York City; Medical Director, Aishel Avraham Residential Health Care Facility, Brooklyn, New York; Chairman of the Board, Association of Orthodox Jewish Scientists

Rabbi J. David Bleich

Rosh Yeshiva, Rabbi Isaac Elchanan Theological Seminary, Yeshiva University; Herbert and Florence Tenzer Professor of Jewish Law and Ethics, Cardozo School of Law, Yeshiva University; Rabbi, Yorkville Synagogue, New York City

Rabbi Mordechai Halperin, M.D.

Director, Falk Schlesinger Institute for Medical-Halachic Research, Shaare Zedek Medical Center, Jerusalem; Editor, *Assia*, Journal of Halacha and Medicine

Lord Immanuel Jakobovits

Chief Rabbi, British Commonwealth of Nations, from 1966 to 1991

Fred Rosner, M.D.

Director, Department of Medicine, Queens Hospital Center Affiliation of the Long Island Jewish Medical Center; Assistant Dean and Professor of Medicine, Albert Einstein College of Medicine, Yeshiva University

Abraham Steinberg, M.D.

Director, Pediatric Neurology, Shaare Zedek Medical Center, Jerusalem; Chairman, Department of Medical Ethics, Hebrew University

Rabbi Moshe D. Tendler, Ph.D.

Rosh Yeshiva, Rabbi Isaac Elchanan Theological Seminary, Yeshiva University; Rabbi Isaac and Bella Tendler Chair in Jewish Medical Ethics, Yeshiva University; Chairman, Department of Biology, Yeshiva University; Rabbi, Community Synagogue of Monsey, New York

FOREWORD

The Raphael Society, Health Care Section of the Association of Orthodox Jewish Scientists (AOJS), sponsored an International Physicians' Conference on Medicine and Halachah (Jewish law), which was held at the Fifth Avenue Synagogue in New York City on January 1–2, 1989. More than 250 attendees participated in this pioneering conference, where it was resolved that future conferences were necessary and desirable.

World-renowned Torah and medical authorities presented papers on subjects spanning the spectrum of medical–halachic dilemmas. Technological advances place us in a maelstrom of new and pressing issues. The subject of acquired immunodeficiency disorders (AIDS) continues to dominate the scientific and secular press. Government intervention, third-party payers, and dissatisfied physicians have focused increasing attention on the need to change the medical system to a monetary cost-containment one no longer concerned with the needs of the "one" but rather with the needs of the societal "many." It is the function of Jewish medical ethics symposia to restore the floundering secular ethic of the day to an even keel.

The content of these proceedings is the basis of this

book. The viewpoints expressed here represent the Torah-
oriented approach to medical ethics as taught in days of old
by the Torah giants such as Maimonides and Nachmanides,
known to scholars and neophytes alike. We are privileged to
have in our generation Jewish medical ethicists of great
renown who bring to these proceedings their wisdom and
insight. Rabbi Lord Immanuel Jakobovits, considered the
father of modern Jewish medical ethics, delivered lectures in
Jewish medical ethics at the Fifth Avenue Synagogue in the
late 1950s and early 1960s. These lectures served as the
beginning of the medical section of the association. Our
American contingent—Rabbis Moshe Tendler and J. David
Bleich—continues to impart the wisdom of the Torah to
succeeding generations of American-trained physicians. Our
Israeli colleagues—Dr. Abraham Abraham, Dr. Abraham
Steinberg, and Rabbi Dr. Mordechai Halperin—remind us
that

> Out of Zion shall come forth Torah, and the word of the
> Lord out of Jerusalem.

Many people participated in the planning of the conference and made these proceedings possible: Drs. Simcha
Ben-David, Marshall Keilson, Susan Schachner, Robert
Schulman, Susan K. Schulman, Mark Singer, Nora Smith,
David Victor, and I devoted long and arduous hours to the
Conference Planning Committee. A special thanks to our
executive director, Joel Schwartz, M.S.W., for his Herculean
efforts not only with this conference but with all the AOJS
activities that he tirelessly coordinates.

"Acharon, Acharon, Chaviv . . ." AOJS is truly for-
tunate to have a member such as Dr. Fred Rosner. One of the
most prolific American writers in the field of Jewish medical
ethics, Dr. Rosner took upon himself the editing of these
proceedings. In addition to serving as Director of the
Department of Medicine at the Queens Hospital Center

Affiliation of the Long Island Jewish Medical Center, and Assistant Dean and Professor of Medicine at the Albert Einstein College of Medicine of Yeshiva University, Dr. Rosner is the Chairman of the Bioethics Committee of the Medical Society of the State of New York, a member and former co-chairman of the Committee on Medical Ethics of the Federation of Jewish Philanthropies, a member of the Professional Advisory Board of the Kennedy Institute for Ethics of Georgetown University, and a member of numerous other prestigious medical ethics committees, including that of Yeshiva University. It is fitting that Rabbi Lord Jakobovits refers to Dr. Rosner as "the leading medical writer on Jewish medical ethics." Dr. Rosner never refuses an AOJS project and attacks each endeavor with a zeal and enthusiasm that is admired by all. *Yashar Kochacha!*

I look forward to the Second International Physicians' Conference planned for May 1990 with the hope that these conferences will facilitate the understanding that—although tremendous progress has been made in the field of biomedical research—true healing is a divine function, and we, the medical practitioners, serve as the Lord's assistants.

Allen J. Bennett, M.D.
Chairman, Board of Governors
Association of Orthodox Jewish Scientists
New York, January 1990

PREFACE

The Rephael Society was founded by Yashar Hirshaut, M.D., late in 1966 in Washington, D.C., as an independent association of Orthodox Jewish physicians and dentists determined to deal with the unique problems facing the observant Jew engaged in the health professions. At about the same time, the Medical–Dental Section of the Association of Orthodox Jewish Scientists (AOJS) was organized in New York City with essentially the same goals as the Rephael Society.

To avoid fragmentation in ongoing efforts to organize Orthodox Jewish health care professionals, the Rephael Society, at the end of 1967, became an affiliate of the AOJS. This affiliation proved mutually beneficial. Therefore, the Washington-based Rephael Society and the New York Medical–Dental Section of AOJS merged to form a new professional group, now known as the Rephael Society, Health Care Section of the AOJS. The merger was approved by a vote of the Board of Governors of AOJS at their annual convention in Monsey, New York, on September 2, 1968.

An active organizational effort converted the largely local programs of the two parent groups of the new Section to national and international programs that serve Orthodox

Jewish physicians, dentists, and nurses, and other Orthodox Jewish health care professionals throughout the United States and Canada. One of these programs was the International Physicians Conference on Medicine and Halachah (Jewish law) held in New York City on January 1 and 2, 1989. This conference was conceived by the then President of AOJS, Allen Bennett, M.D., and implemented by a dedicated group of members of the planning committee (see Dr. Bennett's Foreword) to whom AOJS is indebted.

The present book represents the Proceedings of the conference at which a variety of important modern medical issues were discussed by prominent rabbis and Jewish physicians from the moral, ethical, and Jewish legal standpoints. I am indebted to my loyal secretary, Mrs. Annette Carbone, for typing most of the individual chapters. I am appreciative of the continual and continuing efforts of Dr. Allen Bennett, now Chairman of the Board of AOJS, and Mr. Joel Schwartz, Executive Director of AOJS. The staff of Jason Aronson publishers are to be congratulated for their diligence and high standards in guiding this book to publication.

Finally, I offer praise and thanks to Almighty God for having given me the ability to edit this most important medical ethics book. May He continue to give me strength and health so that within a year we may see the publication of the Proceedings of the Second AOJS International Physicians Conference on Medicine and Halachah, which was held in New York City on May 6 and 7, 1990.

Fred Rosner, M.D.
New York City
June 1990

1

THE ROLE OF JEWISH MEDICAL ETHICS IN SHAPING LEGISLATION

Lord Immanuel Jakobovits

When I am asked to give a ruling on a question of Jewish medical ethics, I act as a rabbi. Even then, more often than not, I do not reach a decision on my own but consult with my *beth din* (Jewish court of law) and others, especially on questions involving life-and-death consequences. But it is as a rabbi that I pronounce the verdict to the questioner.

When I write or speak on Jewish medical ethics, however, my aim is not to give decisions, or to exercise my rabbinic prerogatives. Rather, I act simply as a purveyor of the material as I find it, trying to present it as best I can, and as objectively as possible. I will convey lenient as well as stringent opinions, usually without taking sides. When I discover consensus among leading authorities, I will so indicate. But when opinions differ, I will present the differing views without injecting my own.

When I specialize in medical ethics, I do not do so as a *posek* (rabbinic decisor). I leave that to the sources and to the acknowledged rabbinic authorities of our time. I merely communicate their verdicts and the reasoning behind them. Thus, when I conduct a regular discussion group of Orthodox Jewish physicians at my home in London every couple of months to discuss current halachic (Jewish legal) problems in medicine, I lay before the group as wide a range of authentic opinions as I can find, but I do not give rulings unless there is a clear preponderance of opinion on controversial issues.

The subject of Jewish medical ethics addresses itself primarily to physicians—naturally, physicians who care to be guided by Jewish law. It tells them how to conduct their practice: what they may or may not do in situations impinging on moral or religious issues. Occasionally, Jewish medical ethics also directs the patient, advising him of the moral stance in the light of Jewish teachings. But in this chapter I will address myself less to physicians and to patients than to rabbis. That is, I will focus on how the authentic teachers of Judaism are to present Jewish medical ethics, how the subject develops from a study of our sources and its application within the Jewish community and even beyond, and how in certain cases we are to try to influence legislation. Specifically, how do we convert our teachings of the Halachah into legislative measures?

SECULAR VERSUS JEWISH MEDICAL ETHICS: A FUNDAMENTAL CONTRAST

There is a basic difference between secular medical ethics—now a popular subject taught in many universities and widely discussed in professional and lay journals—and Jewish medical ethics. Secular medical ethics seeks to turn ethical guidelines or rules of conscience into law, into legislation or codes of conduct. Ethical insights or judgments are gradually being distilled into legislative measures or professional rules. In the secular realm, the law is the product of moral intuition or consensus.

Jewish medical ethics operates in reverse. Out of legal verdicts presented as law in legislation or rulings we distill the ethical guidelines and principles responsible for the legal judgments. Jewish medical ethics *derives* from legislation; it does not *lead* to legislation, or at least not commonly so. For us, the legislative rulings have been given as Halachah, or legal norms, and we then have to extrapolate or enucleate the ethical rules and moral principles from them. It is important to bear this distinction in mind in order to understand the rest of this chapter.

I will, of course, further discuss our relationship with legislation, particularly how and where we should endeavor to use our ethical commitments—in turn derived from our halachic commitments—to influence modern legislation. Obviously, in the first instance we have to deal with legislation for Jews or in a Jewish society (i.e., with legislation in the Knesset, the Israeli Parliament). Only then can we turn our attention to non-Jewish legislatures, determining whether and how we should use our influence to bear on general non-Jewish legislatures, such as the United States Congress, or Parliament in Britain. As Jewish citizens, we clearly have certain moral obligations, perhaps even halachic duties, at least to contribute to the public debate on moral issues in medicine, but perhaps also to apply our influence in the formulation of legislation. These are, of course, two entirely distinct situations: the Jewish imperatives in Israel may be altogether different from those appertaining when Jews constitute a small minority. In both cases, I want to use whatever personal experience or attitude I have, regarding both involvement and noninvolvement.

ISRAELI LEGISLATION:
AUTOPSIES AND ABORTION

In principle, I have always opposed the idea of seeking to enforce halachic discipline in Israel by way of Knesset legislation, thus subjecting the majority of Israel's citizens— secularist as they sadly are—to "religious coercion." By and large, I seek to minimize efforts by the religious minority to impose its commitments on the nonobservant majority by legislation. As a rule, this can only further alienate the secular majority from the religious minority and their beliefs. But there are bound to be certain basic exceptions.

One obvious exception concerns the protection of the vital interests of the religious community. Sometimes this cannot be done except by legislation. One notable example is autopsies. This subject has brought about enormous conflicts and collisions in Israel. It has sparked riots in the streets and has caused governments to fall. Of course, the problem is particularly acute in Israel because non-Jews who may not object to autopsy are simply too few to provide the bodies needed for medical education and medical research. Sometimes autopsies are needed to establish the cause of death. This is particularly true in cases in which new treatments or medications have been applied, or in which hereditary factors may be involved. Religious qualms, where they exist, could be assuaged in most cases simply by insisting on family consent.

I have been continuously involved in this issue, both in Israel and in the United States, for the past twenty or thirty years, and I have always maintained that in insisting on family consent, Israel should at least demand no less than what is demanded by any other civilized society in which such consent is required. I am not referring here to medical examiner (coroner) cases, in which suspicion of foul play must be explored or established in an autopsy. Nor am I referring to the small number of cases in which only an autopsy would help to remove a potential hazard to others, such as cases in which a new medical treatment had been applied or in which genetic factors were suspected as the cause of death. Outside this very narrow range of cases, every civilized country, including the United States, Great Britain, and France, requires that permission be obtained from relatives before an autopsy is performed, unless the deceased himself gave consent before his death.

In Israel, hospitals were originally in effect permitted to claim custody of bodies, and free to carry out autopsies without obtaining relatives' consent. When consent is required, abuses are avoided and religious scruples are respected for those to whom the honor of the dead is supremely precious, those who would not easily consent except by a rabbinic verdict (which may well be permissive in certain circumstances). To legislate the requirement for family consent for autopsies is relatively easy. It results in neither religious coercion nor irreligious violation of human rights as claimed by religious citizens.

The second major issue in Israeli legislation to provoke massive conflict is at the opposite end of the spectrum of human life. This is the issue of abortion. Here again, I have been involved for many years in the public debate on this highly contentious issue, including discussions with the religious parties, lecturing to the Israel Medical Association, and publishing my views in the *Jerusalem Post*. In this case, I believed that precise legislation was vital, but that its presentation was all-important. In light of the fact that the majority of Knesset members do not share our respect for Halachah, it was imperative that legislation on a subject such as abortion be presented in a manner that would be persuasive to them and lead them to consider our concerns.

It seems strange that for a long time there was absolutely no agitation on abortion in religious circles. Even the Agudah did not raise the matter until the mid-1970s. It had evidently been of no major concern to them or to the other

religious parties. Why did abortion not figure prominently
on the religious agenda? The reason is very simple. Abortion
did not affect the religious community. No one forced
anyone to have an abortion, so the religious community felt
no need to seek legislation on the subject. As a result,
abortion legislation—liberal as it was in practice—was for
many years altogether neglected.

My lecture to the Israel Medical Association was delivered on May 19, 1970. Its main focus was Jewish medical
ethics in general, but I had to make a reference to abortion,
which was an acutely painful subject in Israel. I asked the
Association for the current statistics on the number of
abortions performed annually. They quoted 40,000 as the
most recent figure. That was twenty years ago! This was
something absolutely catastrophic for the security of Israel,
quite apart from halachic considerations. The *pikuach nefesh*
(survival) of the Jewish people itself was at stake. We had by
now wiped out before birth, smothered in their mothers'
wombs, something like 2 million potential Israelis who
would have been born and bred as perfectly healthy children.
All this as a result of liberal abortion laws and practices. For
all intents and purposes, abortion was available on demand,
or virtually on demand. In fact, the Israeli abortion rate is
proportionately about twice as high as the British rate, and
Britain has very liberal abortion laws. Surely this is intoler-
able, not merely for religious reasons but also for national
ones. Had Israel eliminated the evil of easy abortion, the
Jewish population would today be well over 5 million
instead of 3 million, and what a difference this would have
made to Israel's security if not to its economy as well! Had
the public battle been fought on these grounds and not
simply on a strictly religious basis, the response might have
been altogether different. The religious element might not
only have carried the day in favor of stricter abortion laws,
but it might also have won greater respect and appreciation
from the population at large.

I use this illustration to show that in terms of legislation what is at stake is not merely the strict demands of Halachah. Of critical importance is the effect that the discipline of Halachah has on the Jewish public in general, on the whole people of Israel. Here we have defaulted and often missed great opportunities. In my letter to the *Jerusalem Post* (published on December 1, 1971), I was particularly incensed by a vicious editorial opposing any amendment to the abortion law, which, the paper argued, would serve only to increase the number of unwanted children in Israel. The editorial contained not a single reference to the national disaster of Israel's Jewish population's having been reduced by 50 percent or more through the neglect of Jewish ethics on abortion. I wrote:

> As a national death-wish with catastrophic consequences, few items can rival your editorial (2 November) in support of the pro-abortion lobby, duly followed by success in the Knesset. . . . It advocates pity for "the unwanted children" by strangling them. Unwanted, one might ask, by whom? Perhaps by you and the vociferous abortionists. But certainly not unwanted by the nation, or by most parents, to whom every child, once it is born, is an infinitely precious blessing, whatever the sacrifice, and least of all by the children themselves, who treasure life whether they were "wanted" or not before they were conceived.

Yet I knew that purely legislative pressure was not the answer, and I took issue with the Agudah when it threatened to leave the coalition over the refusal to tighten the law by new legislation. I continued in my letter:

> If I have nevertheless urged the Agudah, and its Council of Sages, not to abandon the coalition over this issue, it is not because I doubt its supreme importance from every point of view, religious and moral as well as national. Rather, scan-

dalous as the present law legalizing rampant abortion is, I do
not believe that legislation by itself will provide the answer.
I agree with you that the amendment would, sadly, not make
much practical difference. Even before the law was liberal-
ized three years ago and abortions for social reasons were
illegal, there were thousands of violations without any
prosecutions.

The ultimate solution to this as to so many other social
problems afflicting our people lies in cultivating a religious
conscience through nurture in the spiritual treasures of our
faith. Where this prevails, parents cheerfully raise large and
happy families, blessed with children who are generally as
immune to the scourges of crime and vice as to the erosion of
assimilation, who preserve their dignity even in physical
deprivation, and who assure Jewish survival by heeding
Rachel's timeless cry, "Give me children, or else I die!"

Knesset legislation can have at least an educational value
in defining what is morally and even socially acceptable, thus
bringing the whole society of Israel gradually closer to
becoming a Torah society.

BRITISH LEGISLATION

Let me now turn to my second major topic: non-Jewish—in
particular, British—legislation. With my elevation to the
House of Lords, I am now a legislator myself, sitting in the
Upper House of the British Parliament. I can vote and I can
contribute to debates if I care to. For me the problem
therefore has a particular immediacy. But in a wider sense,
the issue challenges every Jewish citizen: To what extent
must he bring his Jewish moral convictions to bear on
society in general and the laws governing it? For myself, I
never asked for this opportunity; but now that I have it, how
do I use it?

First of all, the major areas of medical ethics legislation clearly deal with items that come under the heading of the Seven Noahite Commandments. For instance, the question of the definition of death, which requires parliamentary legislation, covers the definition of murder, and this is one of the Seven Commandments. Indeed, for non-Jews this commandment is (in the Jewish view) particularly rigid in its scope. Thus, the Talmud interpreted the Noahite reference to bloodshed—"Whoso sheds the blood of man, by man shall his blood be shed" (Genesis 9:6)—to include the shedding of man's blood "inside man" (i.e., the killing of an unborn child). In any event, the law itself demands that we define life, death, and the point at which death sets in—and for all this we need legislation. We should endeavor to ensure, as best we can, that non-Jews fulfill the Seven Commandments incumbent on all humans, and for that legislative enactments are required.

Beyond murder, the laws on incest and adultery—equally enjoined on non-Jews under the heading of immorality—call for legislation on, for instance, artificial insemination and in vitro fertilization, to determine the identities of the father, the mother, and the blood relatives. On all these issues, the Torah requires us to express our views and to promote their universal acceptance. Where the opportunity exists, we should obviously reinforce through legislation these principles of morality.

The examples already given cover such diverse and important areas as the definition of death, abortion, artificial insemination and fertilization, and derivatives of these practices, such as semen freezing or egg donations. Strict as these universal laws may be, non-Jews may also be covered by the exemptions granted to Jews in special circumstances, such as the sanction to destroy an unborn child if the continued pregnancy would threaten the life of the mother, at least according to Tosafot. Such exemptions should also be reflected in whatever legislation we advocate or support for the nation at large.

Let me give an illustration of my personal experience during this past year in the House of Lords. I took part in a debate on what was called the "Infant Life Preservation Bill." The subject was abortion, and I spoke as a Jew. Indeed, I was elevated in order to bring a Jewish voice to bear on public opinion and public legislation. In Britain, as in the United States *Congressional Record*, every word spoken in Parliament is recorded and then published the next morning. In the course of my contribution, as it appears in the *Hansard* transcript, I said:

> The debate is wide-ranging and apparently, from what I can make out, to some extent the House is divided in opinion on denominational lines within Christianity. Therefore perhaps it is just as well that I should add some thoughts from another perspective. . . .
>
> The tradition that I represent is fairly liberal on the subject of abortion. Judaism regards neither full human status as commencing from conception, nor the destruction of a human fruit before birth as murder. Nevertheless, we deem prenatal human life as very sacred indeed, and would sanction its deliberate termination only in very exceptional cases of grave medical urgency, including some serious psychological threat, provided these indications are absolutely genuine and independently ascertained.
>
> We are less concerned with the stage of gestation than with the motives; if the indications especially for the safety of the mother are urgent enough we may contemplate a termination even after 28 weeks, and if they are not compelling or purely social we would object even under 18 weeks. Obviously the objections increase with the development from conception to birth. . . .

I then dealt with "mental health" as the usual, but quite fraudulent, medical indication for the vast majority of abortions carried out in Britain:

Let me turn attention to the norm—the great majority of cases where abortions are carried out quite legally in this country. I believe that even worse than the law plainly permitting abortion on demand, on social grounds, is the law pretending to prohibit this but in practice using mental health as a legal subterfuge to camouflage what the Prime Minister very recently in a different context so strikingly called "sociological alibis."

The official government statistics for 1986 tell us that out of nearly 135,000 legal abortions in England and Wales "with mention of a medical condition," almost 132,000 were registered as due to "mental disorders." Our population surely cannot be all that mentally sick or at risk!

Clearly in the vast majority of cases doctors resort to this euphemism simply because they would not otherwise remain within the bounds of legality. Some of the evidence in the report submitted to the Select Committee frankly admits this. For instance, the memorandum by the Royal College of Psychiatrists explicitly mentions "termination on medical and social grounds," while the memorandum by Dr. Barbara Jacobs likewise refers to abortions performed for "social reasons" or in "social circumstances."

Such semantic abuse of "mental health" as a cloak for personal convenience or social preference perverts the intent of the law and imposes unacceptable forms of misrepresentation on doctors. It makes a mockery of the law itself and brings it into disrepute. The law should not encourage such terminological inexactitudes, to use another Prime Minister's celebrated phrase.

On the specious argument that the woman should have the right to do with her own body as she pleases, I added that this was quite unacceptable in the Jewish view:

Wherever the limit is set, whether at 28, 24, 20, or 18 weeks, the opposition will always use the well-worn argument that

a woman should have a right over her own body. . . .
There is a double fallacy in this. First, the germinating life
inside her is not exclusively part of her body; it is equally the
flesh and blood of the father who sired it. Moreover, even her
own body is not her property that she can dispose of at will.
We are not the owners but only the custodians of our bodies,
charged to protect and preserve them. The argument against
arbitrary abortions has nothing to do with feminism or male
chauvinism, and the public should be disabused of any such
fallacious notion.

Finally and perhaps most expressive of the Jewish
attitude, I returned to the wider moral issue at stake:

Above all, there is an overriding moral principle at stake here
which is all too often overlooked. The common reasoning is
that the alternative to legal abortions is to encourage back-
street abortionists. It never seems to occur to our vociferous
advocates of easy abortions that there is a third option to
prevent unwanted pregnancies, and that is to train people to
act responsibly, to exercise some self-discipline, and to
cultivate a moral conscience. Instead we are encouraging
what I can only call a credit-card morality—enjoy yourself
now, and pay later.

It is an insult to the moral fibre of countless young
people, and to the moral potential of all of them, to suggest
they are bound to surrender to temptation and cannot resist
it. I have the same complaint about the AIDS publicity
campaign. Surely the only answer to the threat of infection is
not the condom, as if self-control were no longer even an
option which ought to be tried or propagated.

Finally, I miss two other basic considerations in the
report. There may be numerous unwanted pregnancies.
However, there are fewer unwanted children. Once they are
born, they often turn out to be the sunshine of their mothers'

lives or else of those desperately seeking children for adoption.

Again, particularly in this age of widespread violence, terrorism, and war, we should remember that any attack on innocent human life, whether on potential life before birth by abortion or on ebbing life before natural death by euthanasia, cheapens all life, erodes the reverence for it and diminishes the worth of all of us. The respect for all life must start with the beginning of every life.

I have provided this account merely by way of illustration. As Jewish citizens, we must contribute to discussions of grave moral concern in the legislative decisions being made for the society in which we live.

NATIONAL LEGISLATURES INVITING JEWISH VIEWS

Often, of course, it is not we who seek to communicate our concerns, our beliefs, and our insights on proposed legislation, but the legislators who turn to us as groups of citizens for advice. From time to time, Jews everywhere face such a situation. When the promulgation of new laws involving basic moral considerations is contemplated, religious leaders and communal spokesmen are often consulted in one form or another, and we want to make sure that such advice given by Jewish spokesmen bears the hallmark of Jewish teachings.

In the United States, for instance, I know of two specific bodies that have invited Jewish views with the intention of formulating official policies on new legislation. One is the President's Commission for the Study of Ethical Problems in Medicine and Behavioral Research, which, in November 1982, issued a very revealing volume called *Splicing Life: A Report on the Social and Ethical Issues of Genetic Engineering With Human Beings*. This commission, which was set up under the auspices of the White House, consulted various agencies, including some very authentic Jewish respondents. The submissions published in that volume are used for legislative purposes by committees especially appointed for this purpose.

Likewise, there is in the United States, under the auspices of the U.S. Department of Health, Education, and Welfare, a group known as the Ethics Advisory Board. This board issued on this particular subject a report called *Ethical Issues in Human In Vitro Fertilization and Research Involving Early Human Embryos*, published in Washington, D.C., in May 1979. This report also had a Jewish input.

These studies make proposals and/or recommendations to the legislatures to investigate the religious, social, and public attitudes toward various areas of moral concern. As custodians of our particular religious faith, we are invited to make representations and are obviously, therefore, charged to give responses that reflect our moral heritage and convictions.

When a similar body was set up in Britain (known as the Warnock Committee and headed by Baroness Warnock) to present proposals to Parliament on new legislation concerning human fertilization and embryology, I was invited to give evidence, first in writing and then orally, before the committee. These submissions were then used in the committee's report, and proposals for legislation based largely on this report will soon be submitted in the two Houses of Parliament. Thus, on three different occasions Jewish opinions were invited on this one subject of in vitro fertilization and were submitted for the formulation of national legislation. Jewish medical ethics, however diluted, thus finds its way into the laws governing the wider society.

Finally, let me cite a third example that goes beyond national legislation. Not long ago I had a letter from Professor Jean Halpern of Geneva, acting for the World Jewish Congress. The congress had received an inquiry from the World Council of Churches in regard to legislation then being contemplated by the European Parliament in Strasbourg. Among the items to be dealt with was "biotechnology." It appeared to the World Council of Churches, as they put it in their letter, that the attempts to promote eugenics under Hitler were relatively benign compared to the implications of the proposed European legislation. That was their view, and they turned to the World Jewish Congress for a Jewish opinion. This inquiry, with details on the proposal, was transmitted to me. In an effort to obtain further details on the proposal, I turned to a British member of the European Parliament, a good friend of mine who also sits in the House of Lords. He put a written question to the European Parliament on this allegation. This written question, as it appeared in print, simply read:

Is the Commission aware of the deep anxiety both by Christian and Jewish leaders over the content of this recent draft directive on the legal protection of biotechnological inventions? Will the Commission undertake to consult with religious representatives on the moral implications of the proposed directive especially as regards genetic experiments involving human life?

The written reply as I received it from Strasbourg read as follows:

The Commission has not to date put forward the proposal of the directive on the legal protection of biotechnological inventions. Such a directive is, however, referred to in the 1985 White Paper on the completion of the internal market and is under preparation within the services of the Commission.

This proposal should not give rise to anxiety among religious leaders particularly as the inventions concerned do not involve experiments on the human body.

The Honourable Member's concerns, therefore, relate not to this proposed draft directive but to wider issues. The Commission is aware of the public concern regarding these matters and is organising a conference entitled "Human Embryos in Research." Religious opinions will be heard.

Here is an example of the phenomenon of legislative bodies—such as the European Parliament, a new factor in legislation—encouraging Jewish concerns to impinge on proposed laws, and thus providing opportunities for Jewish input.

EXPERIMENTS ON DEAD FETUSES

My most recent inquiry concerned the use of fetal material for experimental purposes. The question concerns only fetuses that have been aborted and are dead. Proposals have been made to use such fetal tissues for experimental purposes. A strict code of practice has been drawn up and is being submitted to various groups—including Jewish ones—for their opinions. I discussed this matter with the *dayanim* (judges) of my *beth din*. We came to the conclusion that, under the very carefully defined restrictions included in the proposed code of practice, we had no objection to the use of aborted fetuses for experimental purposes, and we so informed the government department dealing with the impending legislation on this subject.

Thus, the situation varies: sometimes we will have restrictive views, and at other times our views are permissive, depending, of course, on the issues raised. Indisputably, however, we have a duty as custodians of what we believe to be the universal moral order as enshrined in the Seven Noahite Commandments, and more extensively in the divinely ordained laws of the Torah, to do our utmost to advance the appreciation and the rule of these moral values.

CONCLUSIONS

Human life is infinitely valuable, and the resultant Jewish teaching is that one minute of life, or any fraction of it, is as precious as the totality of life because infinity cannot be divided. For this reason we are opposed to any deliberate form of euthanasia or the hastening of death. To conclude now as I started, this is not only an individual question, a principle affecting every single life; it is a question of our nationhood as well. As Jews, at any time in our history we could have won release from our suffering, from our martyrdom, from our persecutions—relief for the asking, had we been prepared to accept a form of national euthanasia. We need merely have agreed to give up our distinctiveness as Jews, and to accept the passport of baptism, in order to be like everybody else. We would thus have enjoyed the same freedoms as all others.

We express this refusal to die an easy national death as an escape from suffering every time we recite the *Hallel* prayer: "Let the Lord sorely chastise me, but not give me unto death" (Psalm 118:18). We believe that we cannot purchase the relief from suffering at the cost of life itself. As a people we have suffered grievously; yet with all the tribulations we have experienced we still pray: "Do not surrender us unto death." So long as there is life, however anguished and debilitated, there is hope for rebirth, hope to enjoy a better life in the future.

Thankfully, we live in an age in which this invincible faith has been vindicated. The rebirth occurred not in some distant previous generation, nor will it occur in the age of our children or grandchildren. In our own time we have witnessed it both nationally—in the restoration of Jewish statehood—and religiously—in the phenomenal revitalization of Jewish life and learning; not only nationally, in fact, but *corporately*, in the existence of Israel as a state, and religiously in the resurgence of the Orthodox Jewish com-

munity on a scale not previously witnessed in the whole
Jewish history.

May we once again become the source of inspiration to
the world at large, so that we may one day see the fulfillment
of what was our first assignment when we were born as a
people—the blessing, the promise, and the challenge received by Abraham, our father, as he was told: "Through
you shall be blessed all the families on earth" (Genesis 12:3).

2

MEDICAL ETHICS: SECULAR AND JEWISH APPROACHES

Abraham Steinberg, M.D.

Moral and halachic (Jewish legal) problems in medicine are as complex as its science and technology; they cannot be analyzed or solved by simple wisdom, intuition, good intention, or benign character. Rather, a thorough comprehension of scientific facts and moral-halachic values and specific rules is required in order to achieve morally and halachically defensible solutions to the complex issues that characterize the practice of modern medicine.

The ethical problems confronting us today are not entirely new; many have been discussed for centuries. Society has long recognized that morality is a fundamental necessity in the practice of medicine. Moral codes and discussions of ethical theory have a long and honored place in both philosophical and medical literature. What is new to our era, however, is the recent accentuation of these problems by reason of their unprecedented expansion both in kind and in degree.

Until very recently, the domain of medical ethics was viewed by the secular world in a relatively narrow focus—

primarily that of physicians' professional obligations to one another and to their patients. In most instances, medicine had little to offer except for humane empathy and sympathy. Thus, the patient–physician relationship tended to revolve around the patient rather than around the illness. This characteristic was combined with an overwhelming measure of paternalism, in which the physician was the central figure, making almost all decisions on behalf of the patient, often without the latter's informed consent.

With the enormous advances in medicine and medical technology in recent years, the paternalistic approach has been further accentuated, combined not infrequently with dehumanization and depersonalization in medical practice. The disease, rather than the patient, has become the major point of interest. An "interesting case" is a severely ill person with an unusual disease; patients have been turned into "cases," numbered in rooms and beds, thus losing their identity as individuals. This tendency has swung the pendulum toward an extreme counterreaction, which places the patient in the center of the picture with overwhelming authority embedded in the concept of autonomy.

There are many more causes of this resistance to medical paternalism. Today, the prevailing ethical approach is an almost automatic assumption by many ethicists and patients that autonomy must always supervene. This approach is strongly promoted by Engelhardt.[1]

Recent Changes

Several radical scientific, philosophical, and social changes have occurred over the last two decades and have overwhelmingly influenced the shaping of current medical ethics:

1. H.T. Engelhardt, *The Foundations of Bioethics* (New York: Oxford University Press, 1986).

1. Science. An unprecedented expansion of scientific advances and medical technological capabilities have greatly augmented the range and complexity of clinical and policy decisions in health care. Biomedicine is undergoing a rapid transformation, in terms of both its perceived goals and the appropriate means by which to achieve them. The tremendous power now in the hands of biomedical science and scientists must be controlled and properly channeled to avoid unwarranted, undesired, and possibly dangerous side effects.

2. Philosophy. There has been a shift in the physician–patient relationship from the primacy of beneficence and paternalism to the primacy of autonomy. This theory, inherited from the Enlightenment, stresses rights of privacy and individual liberty. Autonomy, self-determination, and the legal right to privacy have become overriding principles.

The result, especially in the last two decades, has been to undermine the 2,500-year-old Hippocratic model of the physician as the benign, authoritarian, paternalistic decision-maker, taking full responsibility for the welfare of the patient.

There are, however, significant flaws in both the autonomy and the paternalism models when applied to a relationship as complex as the medical relationship. The philosophical critique of these models, based on contextual, existential, and conceptual dimensions, was recently summarized by Pellegrino and Thomasma.[2] They propose a third theory based on beneficence—that is, on acting for the good of the patient, and on virtue. This theory is also imperfect, however, and may prove difficult to apply in a pluralistic society.

Thus many thinkers have come to realize that no single

2. E. Pellegrino and D. C. Thomasma, *For the Patient's Good* (New York: Oxford University Press, 1988).

principle, including the principle of autonomy, can predominate absolutely in healthcare ethics.

3. Society and Economics. A marked change in modern medical ethics has occurred due to the influence of the greater involvement of the public at large in medical decision-making processes, and the increased primacy of economic considerations in individual and policy decisions regarding health and medical care.

Taken together, these social, philosophical, and scientific changes have resulted in a significantly different societal role for medical research and clinical application, a shift in the position of the physician, and a change in the relative role of the physician and the patient in the complex relationship between them. These changes have been paralleled by a wide range of new and unprecedented medical–moral dilemmas.

Thus the rapid and drastic changes in several spheres of modern life, as just described, have created the need for, and indeed have forced into being, the newly formed field of bioethics.

Medical ethics has become a field of multidisciplinary approaches and endeavors, combining knowledge and methods derived from theology, moral philosophy, law, social sciences, life sciences, and various branches of the humanities in order to encompass and enhance the comprehension of the many and complex ethical issues in modern medicine.

We have entered a post-Hippocratic era whose future is uncertain, one in which there is serious question about whether the medical profession will ever again be united under a common set of moral commitments. The task before the profession today is one of reconstruction—building a new code of ethics based on elements from the past that are still viable, and discarding those that are not.

THE JEWISH APPROACH TO MEDICAL–ETHICAL DILEMMAS

Jewish ethics were set forth more than 3,000 years ago, and have been tested and reconfirmed throughout the long history of the Jewish people. The methods, deliberations, values, and principles of this system, as well as their application to patients and physicians, are deeply rooted within observant Jews.

Jewish halachic literature, particularly contemporary work, is filled with ethical dilemmas in medicine. Over the past three decades many books and periodicals have been published that are entirely devoted to Jewish medical ethics.

In the sense of normative Jewish law and philosophy applied to practical medical issues, Jewish medical ethics are characterized by and distinguished from secular medical ethics in at least four aspects.

1. Range

General medical ethics deal with diverse subjects. Jewish medical ethics deal with all these and many more subjects that are halachically of no less importance. Examples of "pure" halachic issues include the proper balance between medical intervention and desecration of the Sabbath and Jewish holidays; medical contraindications for circumcision; the special problems of a *cohen* (priest) as a patient, a physician, a visitor of the sick, or an employee in a hospital, and the prohibition against his contact with the dead; kashruth (fulfillment of dietary rules) of medications and food for the sick; and medical interventions in menstruating women (rules of *nidah*).

2. Underlying Principles

Many of the Jewish moral and legal principles and rules have significant bearing upon the practice of medicine. It is worthwhile to mention a few pertinent fundamental principles, since major differences exist between secular and Jewish moral theories concerning medical–ethical issues:

• Judaism ascribes to commitments, obligations, duties, and commandments rather than to rights and pure hedonism. Beneficence and altruism are promoted over mere nonmaleficence. Current Western pluralistic society promotes the concept of happiness and pleasure as a goal, whereas Judaism views it only as a means to achieve higher moral standards.

• The physician–patient relationship is viewed by Judaism as a covenant, in contrast to the notion of a relationship between freely contracting individuals. This approach is also in sharp contrast to the 1980 revised statement of the American Medical Association's *Principles of Medical Ethics*,[3] which bases the patient–physician relationship on the model of a contract. It states that "A physician shall in the provision of appropriate patient care, except in emergencies, be free to choose whom to serve, with whom to associate, and the environment in which to provide medical services." In Judaism, on the other hand, there is an obligation upon a physician to *always* extend help to those in need of medical services. According to Judaism, the physician is God's messenger in healing people in need. Therefore, the motivation of a physician is geared toward more and better knowledge in order to glorify God in this world; in this way the physician can best fulfill his or her duties to others in need.

• Most educators in the field of bioethics agree that the

---

3. R. M. Veatch, in *Journal of the American Medical Association*, vol. 245 (1981), pp. 2187–2189.

purpose of teaching bioethics should not be to increase humanitarianism. It is a desired result but not an a priori goal. This approach is in sharp contrast to the teaching of Jewish ethics, including Jewish medical ethics. In Judaism the dictum is "To learn in order to perform," meaning that the major aim of the study of Jewish law and ethics is to act accordingly.

One of the most significant differences between current secular and Jewish medical ethics concerns the principle of autonomy. Current general medical ethics has overwhelmingly shifted the focus of decision making from the physician to the patient, thus ascribing the primacy of autonomy in the physician–patient relationship to the patient. The principle of autonomy has become absolute, taking precedence over all other values, including life and beneficence.

It is pertinent to cite some of the critique of this approach by Pellegrino and Thomasma.[4] They suggest that the practical question in clinical decisions is not whether or not we have a right to autonomy. We most certainly do. Rather, the question focuses on the proper exercise of autonomy. Do we have a right to exercise autonomy when the decision we wish to make is not morally good? Are we free to make morally wrong decisions? Have we lost a common consensus on morals to such a degree that there is no longer any community of values? Are there any values in common other than autonomy? By promoting autonomy to the extreme, overriding power, are we not promoting a degradation of moral life and principles? Does this approach not educate to amoral, or even immoral, life? Can a society survive such radical pluralism, such a lack of shared values?

Engelhardt[5] argues that full freedom and autonomy must be guaranteed, even if these qualities appear wrong-headed or downright offensive and evil to others, in order to

4. Op. cit.
5. Op. cit.

maintain a peaceable society. The right of autonomy in this libertarian view takes precedence over the good. This retreat to private morality eventually leads to a moral atomism in which each individual's moral beliefs and actions—unless they disturb the peaceable community—are unassailable. Moral debate thus becomes futile, since each person is his own arbiter of right and good. The traditional notion of ethics as reasoned public discourse in search of the common good is discarded.

Pellegrino and Thomasma[6] argue that the approach advocated by Engelhardt is wrong, and that autonomy cannot and should not overrule all other values. In their view, an ethic based on beneficence more fully embraces the nuances of the patient's best interests.

Judaism ascribes to a higher order of moral conduct, which obligates the individual and society. Autonomy as a concept of respect for others is highly valued and demanded. However, autonomous decisions that do not comply with the required moral standard are overridden by higher moral values, as determined by the Halachah and the value system that govern the life of each individual, patient and physician alike.

Judaism restricts the notion of autonomy to actions that are morally indifferent. Where conflicting values arise, each individual is bound to act in accordance with a high standard of normative moral conduct in order to achieve self-fulfillment. Thus, everyone is duty bound to act according to that standard and to relinquish his temporary wishes. Therefore, in medical situations that involve ethical conflicts, the solution is based on the appropriate Jewish law that governs both the physician and the patient. This approach can be termed a *moral–religious paternalism* as opposed to the Hippocratic *individual–personal paternalism* of the physician.

---

6. Op. cit.

Enhancing individual freedom to the point of destroying moral values in medicine cannot be considered the best solution to complex ethical dilemmas in medicine. We need a set of common and shared values that both the patient and the physician will obey, and this is what Judaism offers those who follow this way of life.

3. Method of Analysis

Whereas general ethics is based on philosophical analysis, Jewish medical ethics is based on halachic analysis. These two fields differ in their mode of discourse and in the relevant cognitive background pertaining to medical problems. These differences typify two divergent approaches to all areas of human endeavor. One of the most important differences in the methods of analysis is the Jewish casuistry approach, which places great emphasis on the specific circumstances and variables of each individual case. This model, which was uniquely expanded by the rabbinic responsa literature of the past several hundred years known as *She'elot U'tshuvot*, is in sharp opposition to the philosophical deductive approach, which considers single major theories and applies them uniformly to all cases.

4. End-Point

Ethics does not supply definite answers because it is a pluralistic approach. MacIntyre[7] has stressed this point: "It is a central feature of contemporary moral debates that they are unsettleable and interminable. . . . Because no argument can be carried through to a victorious conclusion, argument characteristically gives way to the mere and increasingly

---

7. A. MacIntyre, "Why is the Search for the Foundation of Ethics So Frustrating?" *Hastings Center Report*, vol. 9 (1979), pp. 16–17.

shrill battle of assertion with counter-assertion." According
to Pellegrino and Thomasma,[8] the search for common
ethical principles to resolve dilemmas that arise from conflicts is fruitless in a pluralistic society. By contrast, religion
gives a finite and decisive answer, although not always one
that is accepted by all members of the community or even by
all authorities of that religion.

In order to achieve the goal of proper conduct in
medical-ethical problems, the Jewish model calls into operation a third party—the rabbi. Thus, optimally, a triad of
patient–physician–rabbi is formed: The physician is obliged
to treat the patient and to offer the best medical advice; the
rabbi is there to advise on the best solution to ethical
problems that may arise; and the patient has the autonomy to
choose his advisors and to make decisions that do not
involve either medical or ethical expertise. In the final
analysis, this triad should reach the best solution of any
complex medical and ethical issue on its own merits and in
consideration of its specific circumstances. The most qualified person makes the decisions relevant to his expertise.
Specifically, factual issues are resolved by the physician, who
is most qualified to decide such matters, while ethical
dilemmas in the treatment of patients must be resolved
according to fundamental moral-religious principles as interpreted by the rabbi. Thus a great measure of the patient's
autonomous decision is in fact abdicated to those who are
best qualified to make the decision.

The differences between Jewish and secular ethical
theories are many and profound. They can be demonstrated
in various spheres of medical practice, some of which
constitute the major topics of this book.

One of the major contentions between the two fields
relates to the different weights attributed to value of life and

---

8. Op. cit.

the principle of autonomy when the two are in conflict. Judaism ascribes a supreme value to life. Therefore, autonomous decisions to destroy life are invalidated. Hence, suicide is morally and legally forbidden; refusal of life-saving treatment is not respected and its use, in fact, is impelled; active euthanasia is absolutely prohibited under all circumstances; abortion is proscribed except for situations in which the pregnant woman's life is endangered. By contrast, secular moral philosophers, for whom the principle of autonomy is the dominant and overriding principle, advocate abortion, the moral acceptability of suicide, refusal of life-saving treatment, and even active euthanasia.

Similarly, secular ethicists strongly advocate the notion of fully informed consent and complete truth-telling to all patients, ignoring possible ill effects of indiscriminate disclosure of information. This approach is based on a radical rejection of paternalism and an exclusive focus on the principle of autonomy. By contrast, Judaism places a higher value on life and beneficence. Therefore, a careful and individualized balance between autonomy and beneficence is demanded. The physician must carefully consider the proper timing, degree, and mode of the disclosure of information. In the final analysis, the physician should favor the good of each individual patient over the general and indiscriminate principle of autonomy.

Hedonism and the acceptance of the overriding power of autonomy have turned homosexuality into a legitimate "alternate life-style." This change in attitude has had enormous ill effects in our era of AIDS. By contrast, Judaism views homosexuality as a crime and demands the eradication of its practice. Thus the current campaign against AIDS through methods of "safe sex," which supports and actually promotes sexual deviations, is in sharp contrast to the Jewish approach, according to which there is a great need for an educational campaign against immoral life-styles.

CONCLUSIONS

These illustrations point out the differences between a rights
ethic and an ethical theory that demands compliance with
higher moral standards. A rights ethic is a minimalist ethic,
based on only one common value—namely the protection of
individual liberties and the sanctioning of any reference or
behavior as long as it does not disturb the peaceable community. This approach disregards all other shared societal
values. In contrast, Jewish ethics subscribe to moral self-
fulfillment through the obedience of moral–religious norms
and requirements commonly shared by *all* observant Jews,
patients and physicians alike.

3

A PHYSICIAN'S OBLIGATION WITH REGARD TO DISCLOSURE OF INFORMATION

Rabbi J. David Bleich

My task is to describe the halachic view regarding the disclosure of information to a patient, apprising him of the terminal nature of his illness. In fact, I am prepared to make two statements on the topic. The first will be very, very brief. In fact, it will be no more than three words. But let me preface those words with a somewhat longer story. This story concerns a rather modern congregation that had established a number of standing committees. Every year, at the annual dinner, the chairman of each of the various committees was called upon to deliver a report. One of the committees was the ritual committee. The chairman was a gentleman of the old school and each year he got up and delivered the same report. The report consisted of two words: "*Men davent.*" Finally, one year he got up and delivered a three-word speech: "*Men davent nisht!*"

My first statement with regard to disclosing information regarding the terminal nature of an illness is extremely simple: "*Men tor nisht*"—It is prohibited! In the second statement I will attempt to elaborate upon the sources from which that conclusion is drawn, and also to modify that statement in some small way.

RABBINIC DISCUSSIONS OF THE PROHIBITION

Contemporary Sources

Let me begin with several contemporary sources that ostensibly deal with somewhat different issues but nevertheless serve to illustrate the focal point of this discussion. The first source is in the last volume of Rabbi Moshe Feinstein's responsa collection.[1] The responsum deals with a situation involving a patient occupying an intensive care unit (ICU) bed. The question addressed to Rabbi Feinstein is whether the patient may be moved to another room because there is now another patient who can derive more benefit from the type of comprehensive and constant care that is available only in an ICU. In addition to discussing a number of other considerations, Rabbi Feinstein remarks that, if in the process of moving the patient from the ICU to another unit the patient may develop anxiety or emotional distress because he recognizes that he is being relegated to less than intensive care due to the fact that his condition has been judged to be terminal, it is prohibited to move the patient from the ICU. Rabbi Feinstein states very clearly that it is forbidden to reveal the terminal nature of an illness to the patient by either word or deed and that this prohibition is grounded in considerations of *tiruf ha-da'at*—a concern that the emotional distress or anguish produced by such a disclosure might

---

1. *Iggrot Mosheh, Choshen Mishpat*, II, no. 73, sec. 2.

foreshorten the brief period of life that is still available to the patient.

A second responsum in the same volume[2] makes the same point, but in somewhat different language. There the question is "How does one treat a terminally ill patient?" The responsum is addressed to a specific situation in which no efficacious therapy is available; the physician has nothing to offer that might be of benefit to the patient. Nevertheless, Rabbi Feinstein counsels that that patient should be given a placebo, some innocuous substance that serves no medical purpose. Rabbi Feinstein reasons that, in order to prevent the patient from becoming despondent, he must be led to believe that he is being medicated. The physician is obligated to occupy himself with the patient, to spend time with him and pay him attention, and to prescribe medication because despondency is most detrimental to the patient's welfare. In the course of formulating this position, Rabbi Feinstein uses an expression somewhat different from that employed in his earlier responsum. Here the concern is not the fear of emotional shock in the form of *tiruf ha-da'at* that is associated with the revelation of a particular item of information that the patient cannot assimilate. Rather, the concern is that slowly, over a period of time, the patient will become aware of the fact that no one is attempting to treat him, that no one is taking him seriously as a patient, and that he has, in effect, been medically abandoned. The result will be a form of despondency or melancholy and that state, in and of itself, is described by Rabbi Feinstein as "the most detrimental harm to the patient."

Evidence demonstrating the existence of the latter phenomenon, one that is far more widespread than situations usually associated with the concept of *tiruf ha-da'at,* can be found in the Torah in a verse that otherwise defies compre-

---

2. Ibid., II, no. 75, sec. 6.

hension. Moses is told to return to Egypt but before returning he took leave of his father-in-law Jethro: "And he said, I will go and return to my brothers in Egypt to see whether they are still alive" (Exodus 4:18). Moses went to Jethro and told him that he must go back to Egypt. Interpreted literally, this verse tells us that Moses wished to see his brethren in Egypt because he wanted to determine whether they were still alive; it had been such a long time since he had seen them that he was unsure of what may have happened to them in the interim. However, if one endeavors to understand this verse literally, it is simply incomprehensible. The Lord had already told Moses to go to Pharaoh in order to redeem the Israelites and to take them out of Egypt (Exodus 3:12). If the purpose of Moses' return to Egypt was to facilitate the redemption of the Jews, then of course they must still have been alive. One cannot redeem people unless they are among the living. And yet, Moses went to Jethro saying that he was not sure whether his brethren in Egypt were indeed still alive. Moses' statement seems to constitute an obvious falsehood. Nevertheless, among the classical commentaries, only the *Orach Chaim*, Exodus 4:18, draws attention to this apparent falsehood.

Rabbi Ben-Zion Firer[3] explains this passage in a very simple manner. Moses was directed to return to Egypt to deliver the divine command to Pharaoh and ultimately to lead the Jews out of Egypt. But Moses was concerned that the Jews would neither believe him nor listen to him (Exodus 4:1). He was afraid that, even if he were to transmit God's instructions, people would not accept them. Scripture confirms that this is what, in fact, did occur. The Jews did not listen to Moses because of their oppression and hard labor (Exodus 6:9). They did not accept his message with alacrity because they believed that redemption was impossi-

---

3. *Panim Mazbirot le-Torah* II (Tel Aviv, n. d.), pp. 24–26.

ble. Their slavery, oppression, and persecution had been so intense and had continued for such a long time that they were in a state of severe despondency. A person who is despondent and melancholic has no desire to live; chronic depression is itself a form of mental illness. For a person in such a condition, life is not really life. When Moses went to Jethro and told him that he must determine whether the Jews in Egypt were still alive, he meant it quite literally. Was there anyone to rescue? Was there anyone to redeem? Did they still desire to live? If Moses' brethren had no desire to live, then redemption would have been an impossibility.

Rabbinic sources emphasize one basic and fundamental point that is crucial to understanding the Jewish approach to the practice of medicine. Insofar as Judaism and Jewish tradition are concerned, not only is every human life of infinite and inestimable value, but every moment of life is of infinite value as well. There is absolutely no hint within Jewish tradition of a notion of a period of life-anticipation that is so brief or so ephemeral as to be morally meaningless. That concept comes from an entirely different system of ethics. It has no place within an ideological or ethical framework predicated upon the teachings of Judaism.

Early Sources

This point is spelled out in clear detail in a number of sources. The first and perhaps the most obvious is the statement of the Gemara, *Mo'ed Katan* 26b, to the effect that an ill person is not to be informed of the death of a relative or close friend lest he become emotionally upset upon receiving the news. The patient is not to be informed because he might experience *tiruf ha-da'at*. Note that the Sages of the Talmud did not say that every terminally ill patient is subject to *tiruf ha-da'at*. They did not say that every patient will die as a result of the shock of receiving this information. They *did* say that there is a cogent and rational fear that disclosure of such information constitutes at least *safek pikuach nefesh* (possible danger to life). For that reason one must refrain from conveying information of this nature.

There is another provision in an entirely different area of Jewish law that, it seems to me, is also predicated upon a concern for avoiding *tiruf ha-da'at*. The concern embodied in the principle "The words of a dying person (*shekhiv mera*) are as if written and delivered," as formulated by the Gemara, *Gittin* 13a, is based upon the fear that if one fails to fulfill the desire of a dying person he may die sooner, even momentarily sooner, than he would have died otherwise. Ordinarily, one cannot transfer ownership of property other than by employing one of the formal modes of conveyance (*kinyan*). Judaism does not recognize disposition of property by means of testament. Hence, if a person wishes to avoid distribution of his property by operation of the laws of inheritance, he must effect some form of *inter vivos* gift. In order to accomplish that end, there must be some form of *kinyan*. However, the Sages carved out an exception to that rule that prevails in certain limited circumstances. In the case of a person suffering from a serious and possibly terminal illness, the Sages declared that the requirement of *kinyan* is to be completely waived. For a *shekhiv mera,* a mere oral declaration is sufficient to effect a transfer of property; the oral declaration in and of itself serves as the conveyance. The Sages were afraid that, on his deathbed, a person might realize that he lacks the capacity to dispose of his estate in the manner in which he chooses, and that this realization could result in mental anguish that might foreshorten his life.

Concern for mental anguish or distress was recognized by early rabbinic authorities (*rishonim*) in a remarkable situation. Rabbi Asher ben Yehiel, known as Rosh, states in his commentary on *Baba Bathra* 9:18 that a person who is being led out in chains to his execution is also categorized as a *shekhiv mera,* and if a person wishes to divest himself of his property under such circumstances, the provision for *kinyan* is to be dispensed with. Rosh cites the position of Rabbi Isaac Alfasi, known as Rif, who declares that dispensation with the provision for *kinyan* applies not only to a patient who is terminally ill and to a person about to be executed, but even to someone who is about to embark upon a sea voyage or a caravan journey. Rosh disagrees with Rif with regard to the latter two cases—that is, with regard to the dispensation applied in the case of a person who is about to embark upon a sea voyage or a caravan trip. Although danger may arise in the course of travel, argues Rosh, nevertheless such travelers cannot be regarded as being in danger at the time they embark upon their journey. Certainly, the concept of mental anguish (*tiruf ha-da'at*) has no meaningful application in such cases since individuals setting out on a journey are not in a debilitated state such that emotional anguish might hasten their death. However, Rosh agrees that these provisions of Jewish law are fully applicable in the case of a person who is about to be executed. Rosh regards the person being led to his execution as being included in the same category as the terminally ill patient.[4]

---

4. Of course, it might be argued that Rosh asserts only that all persons experiencing imminent danger are to be treated in an ·identical manner; the concept of *lo plug* [no exceptions] might be invoked in justifying such a rule—i.e., many rabbinic edicts are universal in nature and do not admit of exceptions even when cogent grounds exist for not encompassing all situations within the ambit of the edict. Accordingly, it might be argued that a rabbinic law designed to ameliorate a specific concern may well apply in all similar cases even though the concern may be entirely absent in those cases. If so, provisions with regard to those facing imminent death may apply not only to the terminally ill but to those facing execution as well. Nevertheless, the case of a condemned prisoner is readily distinguishable from that of a terminally ill patient and there is no talmudic evidence indicating that the Sages sought to treat both cases in an identical manner because of considerations of *lo plug*. The class of the terminally ill is quite different and much narrower than the broader class of persons facing imminent death, and talmudic references are to the former rather than to the latter. Since Rosh extends this principle to the condemned prisoner despite

Let us analyze the implications of Rosh's position. In the case of a person about to be executed, we are not confronted with a situation involving a person suffering from a terminal illness. The condemned prisoner does not suffer from any debilitating malady. Nevertheless, according to Rosh, since he is about to be executed, rabbinic legislation places him in the same category as a person who is dying of a terminal and debilitating illness. What can the concern possibly be? The person being led to his execution, although he may be shackled in chains, is, as yet, entirely healthy. Once the executioner begins discharging the duties of his office, however, this individual has no chance whatsoever of surviving. The concern must be that, even in instances of death by execution, the process of dying may be completed speedily or it may be prolonged over a somewhat protracted period of time. Apparently, Rosh reasons that if the condemned prisoner were to become emotionally upset, agitation might hasten his death, even though death occurs by means of execution. For that reason, the condemned prisoner is regarded as being within the parameters of the category of *shekhiv mera*—that is, a person whom one dare not excite or cause to become agitated because his death may thereby be hastened.

There is another source that employs somewhat different nomenclature in expressing an identical concern. The Gemara, *Horiyot* 12a, describes the case of a person who is about to embark on a journey and wishes to know whether he will return safely or whether early demise will prevent his return. The Gemara suggests that the would-be traveler retire to a dark place and observe whether or not his shadow casts a second shadow. If his shadow also casts a shadow, he

---

the absence of substantiating talmudic evidence and without explicit reference to the principle of *lo plug*, it certainly appears that he regarded that case to be entirely analogous to that of the terminally ill person, i.e., he presumably regarded *tiruf ha-da'at* to be a cogent concern even in the case of the condemned prisoner.

may be assured that he will return; but if his shadow does not cast its own shadow, he has reason to fear that he will not return. The Gemara immediately qualifies this by remarking that the procedure is not to be recommended because the person attempting this form of divination may become upset, and as a result his "luck" (*mazal*) may be spoiled. Rashi explains that the Gemara's concern is that the shadow test is not foolproof; it is possible that a person may not cast a double shadow but yet return from his journey in perfect safety. Nevertheless, since the traveler fails to observe a double shadow he may become disturbed or upset, and the resultant agitation may itself lead to disastrous consequences. Quite obviously, the concern is to avoid a situation in which a person may become overly apprehensive because that type of mental stress can only have a deleterious effect upon a person's general health and well-being.

There is also a talmudic source that speaks of despondency in comparable terms. The Gemara, *Nedarim* 40a, states that one should not visit a sick person either in the first three hours of the day or in the last three. If one wishes to visit a sick friend or relative, one should do so during the mid-portion of the day. Why should one not pay a sick call during the early morning or late afternoon hours? Because during the first three hours of the day the patient appears to be fresh and relatively healthy. As a result, the visitor will not be prompted to pray for a speedy and complete recovery on behalf of the patient because he will think that prayer is unnecessary. During the last three hours of the day the patient seems weaker and his medical condition appears to have deteriorated. As a result, the visitor may be led to think that there is no hope and hence he will not pray on behalf of the patient. Clearly, then, the concern of the Sages extended beyond disclosing negative information to the patient himself. They counseled even against creating a situation in which negative information is imparted to someone other than the patient because they recognized that despondency,

even of friends and relatives, can have a negative effect upon
the patient. Even if despondency is not contagious, which
may well be the case, it has a negative effect in that it causes
relatives and friends to despair of divine mercy and hence to
abandon hope and abjure prayer.

There are at least two sources that explicitly discuss
divulging the diagnosis of a terminal condition to the
patient. The Midrash, *Kohelet Rabbah* 5:6, comments upon
the biblical narrative that tells of the visit of the prophet
Isaiah to King Hezekiah when the latter was ill. God
instructed Isaiah to inform Hezekiah that the latter was
terminally ill and would not live. The prophet dutifully
discharged his mission. Isaiah visited Hezekiah and delivered
the message as charged by God and also admonished
Hezekiah to give his family final instructions because death
was imminent. The Midrash informs us that Hezekiah
reproved the prophet saying, "Customarily, when one visits
the sick, he says, 'May Heaven have mercy upon you.' A
physician who visits [a patient] tells him, 'This you may eat
and that you may not eat. This you may drink and that you
may not drink.' Even if [the physician] sees that [the patient]
is about to die he does not say to him, 'Leave a testament to
your household' lest the [patient's] mind faint." One is
supposed to pray for the patient and give him a blessing. A
visitor tells the patient that God will help, and gives advice
with regard to diet: This food you may eat, but do not eat
other foods. Drink this liquid, but not some other beverage.
And even if the physician sees that the patient is about to die,
he does not tell him, "Write your last will and testament
because you are about to die." "Why, then," queries
Hezekiah of Isaiah, "did you instruct me to put my affairs in
order because I will not live?" Had God not specifically
commanded Isaiah to deliver that message, Isaiah would
indeed have been remiss in informing Hezekiah that he was
about to die. The concern embodied in that rebuke, the
Midrash tells us, is a concern for *tiruf ha-da'at,* "lest the mind

faint"; i.e., if a patient suffers distress and anguish, that emotional state may itself cause the foreshortening of his life.

Another incident recorded in the Bible is understood by some commentaries in precisely the same way. As recorded in II Kings 8:7–10, Ben-Haddad, the King of Aram, became sick and sent a messenger, Azael, to Elisha. The messenger was to pose one question: Would Ben-Haddad recover from this illness? Elisha informed the messenger Azael that, in fact, Ben-Haddad would die, but he instructed Azael to tell the king, "You shall surely recover." Ralbag, commenting on this verse, indicates that Elisha's concern was precisely a concern for *tiruf ha-da'at,* or mental anguish. Elisha's concern was based upon the very real possibility that the shock of receiving a true response—namely, a prediction of impending death—might in and of itself serve to trigger termination of the life of the patient.

CONTEMPORARY ARGUMENTS FOR DISCLOSURE

Both the Sages of the talmudic period and the early talmudic commentators were extremely clear in formulating their position against divulging the diagnosis of a terminal illness. In contemporary times, four arguments have been presented in support of a policy that is diametrically opposed to the negative view regarding full disclosure that is reflected in rabbinic sources. Two of those arguments are medical or scientific in nature and two can be categorized as ethical or moral in nature. I will first list those arguments and then discuss them each in turn.

The first argument consists of a simple denial of the phenomenon of emotional distress as a life-shortening factor. The concern of *Chazal* for *tiruf ha-da'at,* runs the argument, is entirely misplaced. Scientifically speaking, *tiruf ha-da'at* is a nullity; it does not exist. Emotional pain and psychological anguish do not really shorten anybody's life. The second argument is based upon a claim that truthful information regarding the condition of the patient, even if the patient is terminally ill, is actually beneficial in a variety of ways. Hence, it is in the patient's best interest to be given full and complete information concerning his condition. Thirdly, the patient has a right to know: How can anyone take it upon himself to deny another human being such basic information—information he is rightfully entitled to receive? The fourth argument is that information can be withheld only by means of some type of subterfuge. Usually, an outright lie of one type or another is required. But a lie cannot be sanctioned because lying is absolutely immoral. Lying is a sin; one has no right to lie even if one believes that the lie is designed to achieve a good purpose.

These are the arguments in favor of full disclosure to the patient that have appeared in the medical and psychological literature. Let me deal with them serially.

Scientific Arguments in Favor of Full Disclosure

As noted, the first argument is that *tiruf ha-da'at,* or emotional trauma that might foreshorten life, simply does not exist. The most prominent, but by no means the only, exponent of that position is Elizabeth Kübler-Ross in her books *On Death and Dying*[5] and *Questions and Answers on Death and Dying.*[6] Kübler-Ross has developed an extremely complex theory regarding the psychology of dying and claims to have identified five distinct psychological stages of dying. She argues that ultimately the patient comes to accept death and does so without adverse effect. Kübler-Ross' scientific objectivity and the validity of her conclusions have

5. New York: Macmillan, 1970.
6. New York: Macmillan, 1974.

been challenged by a number of her colleagues,[7] and other researchers have reported markedly different findings.[8] Nevertheless, *arguendo,* I am perfectly willing to accept as absolutely true everything that Kübler-Ross has said, but not more than she has said. Dr. Kübler-Ross conducted experiments involving some 200 subjects. I am perfectly willing to grant her the benefit of any possible doubt, and to concede that the five stages she has identified and labeled constitute an accurate report of the phenomena observed in every one of her 200 subjects. I am also willing to concede that there were no adverse physical effects in any one of those 200 patients. Having done so, I nevertheless find no contradiction in her reports to anything found in rabbinic literature. In examining the words of the Gemara, *Mo'ed Katan* 26b, one should note that the Sages expressed concern "*lest* the patient suffer mental anguish"; in other words, they were concerned about the *possibility* of inducing mental anguish by disclosure of information. They did not contend that this result would obtain in all cases, or even in the majority of cases. They contended only that it may occur in some cases; they did not even hint at how small that minority of cases might be. All forms of inductive reasoning fall short of ultimate proof and demonstration because one cannot examine every possible case. Kübler-Ross has shown, at best, that there were no adverse effects in two hundred patients. Who knows what might happen in the case of the two-hundred-and-first patient?

At least one contemporary study does record and con-

---

7. See R. Schultz and D. Aderman, "Clinical Research and the Stages of Dying," *Omega*, vol. 5 (1974), pp. 137–143; and R. Branson, "Is Acceptance a Denial of Death? Another look at Kübler-Ross," *Christian Century* (May 7, 1975), pp. 464–468. See also *Time* (Nov. 12, 1979), p. 81.

8. See J. M. Hinton, "The Physical and Mental Distress of Dying," *Quarterly Journal of Medicine*, vol. 32 (1963), pp. 1–21; and K. A. Achte and M. L. Vaukkonen, "Cancer and the Psyche," *Omega*, vol. 2 (1971), pp. 46–56.

firm the phenomenon of emotional trauma associated with being informed of an unfavorable diagnosis. It is noteworthy that this fact is conceded by physicians who nevertheless argue for divulging such information to the patient. In an article entitled "Should the Doctor Tell the Patient that the Disease is Cancer? Surgeon's Recommendation,"[9] Victor Gilbertsen and Owen Wangensteen advocate full disclosure. They specifically discuss the question of whether or not one should disclose a diagnosis of cancer to the patient, and they cite statistics that, in their opinion, augur in favor of disclosure. Four percent of surgical patients who received such information became emotionally upset upon learning the nature of their affliction and remained so throughout the course of their illness. Only 4 percent suffered emotional distress and manifested that emotional distress during the entire course of the illness. How many more suffered emotional distress but did not manifest symptoms of distress during the entire course of the illness is not stated. But at least 4 percent *did* manifest emotional distress—and did so until they died! I submit that, if the life of every individual is precious, and if every moment of that life is of infinite and inestimable value, 4 percent is a very, very high rate of incidence. If we are dealing with even only 4 percent who experienced the phenomenon of *tiruf ha-da'at,* statistically that phenomenon is extremely significant; and our Sages certainly had ample reason to make their concern known to us and to make that concern an integral consideration in determining how one is to relate to a terminally ill patient.

At least one source advances the view that full disclosure of information may actually be beneficial to the patient. In an article published in the *British Medical Journal,*[10] Jean

---

9. In *The Physician and the Total Care of the Cancer Patient* (New York, 1962), pp. 80–85, a collection of papers presented at a symposium sponsored by the American Cancer Society.

10. March 21, 1959, pp. 779–783.

Aitken-Swan and E. C. Easson claim that, at least for some patients, disclosure of even the bleakest prognosis serves either to eliminate fear and anxiety or at least to significantly reduce these feelings. The same authors indicate that other benefits are attendant upon this type of disclosure. Presumably this means that, in the case of some patients, the result of full disclosure is a lesser degree of danger of *tiruf ha-da'at*. As will be shown later, the exceptions that these authors have reported are paralleled in at least one rabbinic source. Such observations in no way negate the concern for *tiruf ha-da'at* as a phenomenon that must be anticipated. At the very most, those studies show that there are some people who may actually benefit from having such information revealed to them. The argument developed in explaining the reaction of these patients is that knowledge, even knowledge of the worst, is easier for them to handle than doubt and uncertainty. Even if this thesis is correct, it does not negate or contradict rabbinic teachings regarding disclosure. Even taking that consideration into account, rabbinic authorities regarded the consequences of *tiruf ha-da'at*, in the cases in which it does occur, as too serious to be disregarded. Any benefit attendant upon disclosure that may be enjoyed by some patients, must be weighed against the serious harm such disclosure may cause others. Therefore, "do not disclose" is the recommended course of action. Since the potential harm of full disclosure involves the foreshortening of human life, the harm outweighs any possible benefit that may result.

I will cite two examples of the phenomenon that evoked our Sages' concern, which I have personally observed in my own "clinical practice" as a pulpit rabbi. Many years ago, a middle-aged attorney was hospitalized and told that he was suffering from diverticulitis, an inflammation in small out-pouchings from the large bowel. One day, I walked into the patient's room to find that this individual, whose spirits had been fine up to that point, was in tears; he was broken and shattered, an emotional basket-case. If ever there was a case of *tiruf ha-da'at*, there it was, in front of my eyes! I asked him what happened; why was he so upset? By mistake, a nurse had left his chart in the room. The patient had glanced at the chart and saw that dreaded word: *carcinoma*. I brazenly told him that I was sure there was some mistake: "I know your condition. I spoke with your doctor. You don't have cancer; you have diverticulitis. Wait a minute. I'll go outside and have a look at your chart." I walked outside and paced back and forth in the hall for 10 minutes, doing absolutely nothing. I came back into the room and said, "I saw your chart. The word *carcinoma* does not appear there." The patient's reaction was, "Rabbi, are you sure? Are you absolutely positive that you checked the chart carefully? I'm so glad!" That is not the end of the story. The man lingered on for 6 or 7 weeks, and on subsequent visits I saw a patient with widely fluctuating moods. On some days he was perfectly cheerful and happy. Those were the days on which he believed the lie I had told him. On other days he was extremely depressed. Those were the days on which he told me, "Rabbi, I know that you were lying. I know that you were not telling me the truth." For the psychologist, here was a perfect case of denial and counterdenial. For the student of Jewish law, here was a perfect example of *tiruf ha-da'at*. While one cannot state with certainty that the patient's death was actually hastened by the knowledge he had inadvertently obtained, that knowledge certainly was not beneficial for him. It assuredly caused emotional trauma, and it is not at all far-fetched to suspect that it may have hastened his demise.

Another example involves a situation that did not involve so serious a condition and that fortunately had a different outcome. An elderly gentleman experienced back pain while walking home from *shul* on *Shabbat,* broke out in a cold sweat, and became extremely pale. No one would have challenged the diagnosis of a possible "heart attack." I assume all physicians would agree that a person manifesting such symptoms ought to be sent to a hospital, put into a coronary care unit, and carefully monitored. This man was in fact sent to the hospital. When I visited him there, he told me that his doctor had informed him that "On a scale of 1 to 10, you had a heart attack that is 0.5." Some heart attacks are more severe than others, but, by definition, a "heart attack" means that there has been some damage to the cardiac muscle. The patient's cardiologist had commendably told the patient the truth but had couched the message in language designed to minimize concern. The next evening I received a telephone call from the man's wife. She had been in touch with a relative who happened to be a cardiac surgeon. The relative spoke to the patient over the telephone and told him, "You will probably need bypass surgery." He then proceeded to spell out in great detail the procedures and risks involved in bypass surgery. When I visited the patient the next day, he was in a terrible state; he was clearly in a state of *tiruf ha-da'at* and for no real reason. Fortunately, the man came home after several days and recovered fully and uneventfully without surgery.

This clearly is a situation in which it was irresponsible for the patient's relative to furnish him with a definitive diagnosis and prognosis. The diagnosis happened to be inaccurate, and the patient was alarmed needlessly. But even if the information had been correct, it should not have been conveyed in so insensitive a manner. This is certainly a very dramatic example of disclosure that did not do the patient any good at all. It is an instance in which one may clearly see the phenomenon of *tiruf ha-da'at*.

This phenomenon also finds scientific confirmation in the medical literature. A famous surgeon, J. M. T. Finney, who for man years served as a professor of surgery at the Johns Hopkins Medical School, publicly testified that his many years of experience had taught him to be selective in accepting patients. The mortality rate among his patients was very, very low. Dr. Finney refused to perform major surgery on any patient who expressed fear with regard to the potential success of the contemplated procedure. Dr. Finney's clinical experience had led him to conclude that fear contributes to a high mortality rate, and he managed to keep the rate among his patients artificially low by accepting only patients who were not afraid.[11]

There is also a report in the psychological literature that serves to demonstrate that hopelessness can be a cause of death in animals. A series of experiments was performed with wild rats that were first confined in a metal cage. They were then forced into a black opaque bag in which they could not move. Later they were removed from the bag and their whiskers were cut off in order to cause loss of stimulation. Finally, the rats were dropped into a water-filled glass jar in which they might swim until they were overcome by exhaustion, but from which there was no escape. The procedure was designed to eliminate all hope of escape and to cause the rats to feel threatened.

A significant number of rats died as soon as they were taken out of the bag even before they were dropped into the water; others died immediately upon being placed in the water. None of the rats survived in the water for any significant period of time. In a control group, however, when hopelessness was eliminated, the rats did not die. The elimination of hopelessness was achieved by repeatedly holding the rats briefly and then freeing them, and by immersing the rats in water for only a few moments on several occasions and immediately removing them from the water. The rats quickly learned that the situation was not hopeless. They became aggressive, tried to escape and swam for much longer periods of time. Many rats in this control group swam for a period of between 40 and 60 hours.

---

11. See W. B. Cannon, "'Voodoo' Death," *American Anthropologist*, vol. 44 (1942), no. 2; reprinted in *Psychosomatic Medicine*, vol. 19 (1957), p. 189.

Clinical tests indicated a slowing of the heartbeat and respiratory rate and lowering of body temperature among the rats that died. Autopsies revealed enlarged hearts distended with blood. Researchers who conducted this experiment attributed the early death of the experimental rats to the overstimulation of the parasympathetic nervous system.[12]

Apparently, the rats in the control group, at least on an instinctive level, still had hope; they anticipated salvation in one form or another. Be that as it may, one is clearly confronted here with a situation in which anticipation of survival, even among animals, contributes to survival, whereas anticipation of death contributes to death. In many cases, such anticipations become self-fulfilling prophecies.

There are other psychological studies that serve to confirm that phenomenon. During World War II a considerable number of unaccountable deaths were reported among soldiers in the armed forces. Those deaths occurred among men who were apparently in good health. In autopsies, no pathology was observed. Deaths occurred not as a result of wounds, but of some other unexplained cause. Deaths are also regularly reported among individuals who imbibe small, definitely sublethal doses of poison and among persons who inflict minor, nonlethal wounds upon themselves. In those cases it is assumed that the sole cause of death is simply the victims' belief in their impending doom.[13]

In a well-known investigation of "voodoo death," Dr. Walter Cannon demonstrated that such deaths are readily explainable and have absolutely nothing to do with black magic. The hex is pronounced, and, as a result, the individual is overcome by profound misery, refuses food and drink, and literally "pines away." The explanation offered is that

---

12. See C. P. Richter, "On the Phenomenon of Sudden Death in Animals and Man," *Psychosomatic Medicine*, vol. 19 (1957), pp. 191–198.
13. Ibid., p. 197.

death occurs as a result of persistent excessive activity of the sympathetic adrenal system. Continuous injection of adrenaline produces a constriction of the blood vessels. The resultant decrease in blood pressure causes blood volume to be reduced until it becomes insufficient for maintenance of adequate circulation. Thereupon, deterioration occurs in the heart and nerve centers. As a result of the damage to the organs necessary for adequate circulation, they become less and less able to maintain effective blood circulation. The result is death.[14] Death occurs even though there is no significant reason for such dysfunctions to have occurred in the first place. Death occurs simply because the patient experiences the fear that he is going to die and this fear itself sets into motion physiological processes that ultimately cause death to occur.

A most eloquent formulation of this phenomenon, written by Louis Thomas, appears in the first volume of the *Journal of Medicine and Philosophy*:

> It is not unlikely that there is a pivotal moment at some stage in the body's reaction to injury or disease, maybe in aging as well, when the organism concedes that it is finished and the time for dying is at hand, and at this moment the events that lead to death are launched, as a coordinated mechanism. Functions are then shut off, in sequence, irreversibly, and while this is going on, a neural mechanism held ready for this occasion, is switched on. . . .[15]

Although the article from which this excerpt is quoted appeared in the *Journal of Medicine and Philosophy*, it certainly is not philosophy, and I doubt that it is medicine. But it is certainly poetically moving and serves eloquently to describe the phenomenon of *tiruf ha-da'at*.

---

14. Cannon, pp. 182–190.

15. L. Thomas, "A Meliorist View of Disease and Dying," *Journal of Medicine and Philosophy*, vol. 1 (September 1976), p. 219.

Ethical Arguments in Favor of Disclosure

Enough has been said in rebutting the medical counterarguments to the halachic concern regarding *tiruf ha-da'at*. Let me turn to the ethical arguments, the first of which is based upon the putative right to know. This, in turn, flows from the concept of personal autonomy—that is, the notion that a person enjoys the right to absolute freedom with regard to himself and to his destiny; hence he is entitled to any and all information with regard to himself that he wishes to obtain. The response to that argument is quite simple: No such right is recognized by Judaism. To the extent that liberty and personal autonomy constitute a value, such value consists of freedom *from*, not freedom *to*. For Judaism, freedom as a moral value is freedom from external constraint. The God-given right to develop one's potential to serve the Lord does not include the right to dispose of one's life and one's body in a manner of one's own choosing.

This concept is expressed most beautifully in the language of Halachah in two sources. One is a responsum of Rabbi Betzalel Stern[16] and the other is in a compendium edited by Rabbi Shlomoh Zalman Braun.[17] In both sources, the specific question involves a father who demands of his son that the latter tell him explicitly and unequivocally the nature of his illness. Both authorities rule in no uncertain terms that, even when confronted with a possible infraction of the commandment to honor one's father, there is absolutely no obligation to disclose this type of information. The responsum authored by Rabbi Stern consists of a lengthy dissertation devoted to a delineation of the parameters of the commandment concerning the honor due one's father and mother. Insofar as the specific question itself is concerned, it might have been addressed in a very brief sentence. The

16. *Teshuvot be-Tzel he-Chochmah* II, no. 55.
17. *She'arim ha-Metzuyanim be-Halachah* 193:2.

request for disclosure of information is tantamount to the father's demanding of his son that the latter do something in violation of a commandment of the Torah; under the circumstances, there is no obligation whatsoever to "honor" one's father. A virtually identical and equally brief statement to that effect appears in the work of Rabbi Braun.

Let me turn to the fourth argument in favor of disclosure—namely, that in failing to provide information, one becomes involved in either a subterfuge or an outright lie. The author who formulates that argument most clearly is Sissela Bok, in her book *Lying: Moral Choice in Public and Private Life*.[18] This argument reflects great concern with regard to the grave sin of "lying." After all, Scripture unequivocally declares, "Keep thee far from a false matter" (Exodus 23:7).

At least two of the early rabbinic authorities who enumerate the 613 biblical commandments—Rabbi Moses of Coucy, *Semak*, no. 104, and Rabbi Isaac of Corbeil, *Semag*, no. 226—do indeed list this admonition as one of the 613 commandments. However, other eminent authorities, including some of the most prominent of those who have compiled listings of the commandments (e.g., Rambam, Ramban, *Ba'al Halachot Gedolot*, and *Sefer ha-Chinnuch*), do not enumerate this scriptural admonition among the 613 biblical commandments. For them, this verse must undoubtedly be understood as interpreted by Abraham Ibn Ezra in his biblical commentary—namely, as an exhortation to the *beth din*. According to Ibn Ezra, the cognitive import of this verse parallels the commandment "In righteousness shalt thou judge thy neighbor" (Leviticus 19:15). Indeed, the concluding phrase of the scriptural verse exhorting against falsehood is "and do not slay the innocent and the righteous" (Exodus 23:7), an admonition that is clearly addressed to the

---

18. New York: Pantheon, 1978.

judicial authorities. Talmudic exegesis of this verse interprets the first part of the verse as also dealing with matters pertaining to a *beth din*. The Gemara, *Shevu'ot* 31a, declares, "From where is it derived that the *beth din* dare not listen to one of the litigants before the other litigant appears? From the verse 'Keep thee far from a false matter.'" Failure to observe that procedure would result in a "false matter"—that is, an erroneous decision. Similarly, the Gemara, *Shevu'ot* 30b, queries, "From where is it derived that a judge should not allow an ignoramus to sit before him? From the verse 'Keep thee far from a false matter.'" An ignoramus who participates in the deliberations of the court is likely to utter nonsense, but in doing so he may sway the judges and cause a false decision to be issued. The rabbinic applications of the verse clearly show that the verse is associated with a commandment to the *beth din*. Rabbi Saadia Ga'on, *Sefer ha-Mitzvot*, no. 22, adduces additional evidence in support of the position that there is no biblical prohibition against uttering a falsehood.

Let me be very precise. I do not wish it to be said that I have made a blanket statement to the effect that lying is permissible. There are other prohibitions associated with various forms of falsehood. There is a prohibition against perjury: "Thou shalt not utter a false report" (Exodus 23:1). There is a prohibition against a *beth din* issuing a false judgment: "Thou shalt not wrest the judgment" (Exodus 23:6). There is a prohibition against lying for purposes of illicit monetary gain: "Neither shall ye deal falsely, nor lie one to the other" (Leviticus 19:11). There is a prohibition against various forms of deception. If one is about to go to the mailbox and another person is in the process of leaving the house, one dare not say, "Wait, I will accompany you." One dare not deceive by pretending to perform an act on behalf of another person when that act is actually being performed on behalf of oneself. Such conduct is a prohibited form of *geneivat da'at*, "stealing another person's mind."

Telling a lie for the purpose of causing pain or anguish to another person is prohibited: "Ye shall not wrong one another" (Leviticus 25:14). The statement that, for some authorities, uttering a falsehood is not forbidden is limited solely to a perfectly innocuous lie that harms no person—in other words, a "white lie" from which no one will suffer financially, physically, or even emotionally. Thus, the area of possibly permissible falsehood is extremely limited.

It seems to me that this controversy regarding the permissibility of an innocuous lie is really the substance of the dispute between *Bet Shammai* and *Bet Hillel* as recorded in the Gemara, *Ketubot* 16b–17a. *Bet Hillel* declare that, under any and all circumstances, one should praise a bride's pulchritude as well as her good qualities and traits by lauding her as beautiful and gracious. *Bet Shammai* in effect ask: What if she is a little bit lame or is blind in one eye? Does one still call her beautiful and gracious? Is it not written "Keep thee far from a false matter"? The Torah commands us not to lie! Elsewhere, in *Kallah*, chapter 10, the Gemara clarifies the position of *Bet Hillel*. *Bet Hillel* is reported as having responded that when the Torah commands "Keep thee far from a false matter," it is in the context of the concluding phrase of the verse, "Do not slay the innocent and the righteous" (Exodus 23:7). Thus it is quite evident that *Bet Hillel* espouse an interpretation identical to that of Ibn Ezra and regard the admonition as being addressed to a court of law commanding them to abjure any form of falsehood that may result in the death of the innocent and the righteous. However, when undertaken for a laudable purpose, such as to avoid causing distress to another, lying is entirely permissible.

Why is it necessary to belabor that point, particularly since there are other circumstances with regard to which *Bet Shammai*—as well as the authorities who maintain that "Keep thee far from a false matter" is one of the 613 biblical commandments binding upon all Jews—would certainly concede that lying is permissible? There is no question that all would agree that lying is permissible for purposes of preserving or prolonging a human life. The point that requires emphasis is this: The majority of early rabbinic authorities maintain that distortion in order to preserve the well-being of another is not a matter of choosing the lesser of two evils. It does not constitute a situation in which the law against lying is set aside or waived because of a higher cause, such as one in which the act is intrinsically a transgression but is sanctioned because of an overriding consideration. Failure to tell the truth for the purpose of preventing distress, or even for the purpose of promoting a sense of well-being, is not at all a transgression and hence does not engender a situation with regard to which a person should suffer any remorse whatsoever.

This statement may be very unconvincing, at least to some. Sissela Bok, for example, would be totally unswayed by this analysis of "Keep thee far from a false matter." It would not impress her at all, and I understand her point of view. I understand her perspective very well because it is endemic to the American mentality. I have many shortcomings; one of them is that, despite my white beard and black hat, I am very much a product of American culture. An American can understand and forgive virtually anything and everything, with one exception: he cannot forgive a lie. If you lie to him, even if it is an innocuous lie, he will never forgive you. He will no longer look you in the eye, and he will not willingly continue to have dealings with you. I know because I suffer from that mentality. I react that way. Moreover, I also believe that there is support in Jewish tradition for such a reaction. King David reacted that way when he said, "He that speaketh falsehood shall not be established before mine eyes" (Psalm 101:7). Even in circumstances in which telling a lie is not an outright transgression, it is certainly distasteful and odious and hence should not be undertaken unless there is a serious reason for doing so. But when there *is* sufficient reason for doing so, there is no reason for feelings of guilt.

Even more significantly, in the situation that we are
addressing, the physician's statement denying the terminal
nature of an illness is not necessarily a lie. It is not a lie for
two reasons. In his commentary on the Bible, Deuteronomy
11:13, Rabbi Bachaya ben Asher of Saragossa remarks that
the power of prayer is so great that it can even nullify a
divine decree and cause a change in the operation of the laws
of nature. To tell a patient that he is not terminally ill does
not constitute a lie. Insofar as Judaism is concerned, there is
no irreversible malady: *Al titya'ash min hapuraniyot*—"Do not
become despondent because of misfortune"; it is always
possible to effect a cure. Rabbi Yechezkel Abramsky, of
blessed memory, once put it to me in a very beautiful way.
He remarked that, in the blessings preceding *keri'at shema*,
we speak of God as a *boré refu'ot*, a Creator of cures. Creation
connotes the generation of *yesh me-ayin*, something out of
nothing. If God is the Creator of cures, then a cure can surely
be created literally "out of nothing." Hence one has no right
to assume that a cure is impossible.

There is yet another reason why telling a patient that he
is not terminally ill should not be regarded as a lie. The
Dutch scholar Hugo Grotius argued that lying is always
forbidden.[19] However, there are many situations in which
everybody concedes that a person ought to lie. An obvious
example is a case in which someone solicits information that
he will use for some nefarious purpose. For example, a
burglar breaks into a house and asks, "Where can I find the
rifle so that I can use it to threaten your life?" Clearly, only
a fool would disclose that information. Grotius argues that,
under such circumstances, dissemblance is not a lie. Since the
would-be malefactor is not entitled to such information in
the first place, denial of that information is not a lie. I have
a rabbinic source for that position, a little book by Rabbi

---

19. *On the Law of War and Peace*, trans. F. M. Kelsey et al. (Indianopolis, 1925),
Book III, chapter 1.

Ya'akov Yecheskel Fisch that was published not long ago entitled *Titen Emet le-Ya'akov* (literally, *Give Truth to Jacob*).[20] The work is devoted to the explication of the virtues of truth-telling, but also contains a series of some seventy-five responsa that should properly be titled *Titen Sheker le-Ya'akov* (literally, *Give Falsehood to Jacob*), since these responsa enumerate a series of leniencies with regard to falsehood. One of the considerations cited in this work in permitting certain forms of falsehood is very similar to that advanced by Grotius, but with one important variation. To take a slightly different example from that of Grotius: Suppose someone calls me on the telephone and asks, "What are you doing?" I happen to be counting my money, but I do not wish to tell the caller what I am doing. May I lie or may I not lie? The author of *Titen Emet le-Ya'akov* argues that this is information to which the caller is not entitled. I have no obligation to disclose the truth. But if I were to answer truthfully, "I don't want to tell you. It's none of your business," the caller would be offended. Accordingly, runs the argument, this is a situation in which it is permissible to withhold the truth "for the sake of peace." This consideration allows falsification even when the truth is innocuous, simply because the interlocutor has no claim to the information that he seeks. *A fortiori*, if a patient is not entitled to certain information because the patient has no claim to information that may lead to *tiruf ha-da'at*, and, for obvious reasons, one cannot very well tell him, "I do not wish to answer," the license to lie is clear and unequivocal. Under those circumstances the "lie" is certainly not to be defined as a falsehood within the parameters of the prohibition of "Keep thee far from a false matter."

Does this mean that there are no exceptions to the principle that a patient should not be informed that he is

---

20. Jerusalem, 1982.

suffering from a terminal illness? On the basis of this
discussion it would seem that there are none. It sounds very
much as if this entire presentation is in the form of what, in
legal circles, would be termed a general denial. The jocular
example of a general denial is portrayed in the situation of an
attorney representing a chicken thief. The defendant is
accused of having stolen chickens. The attorney goes to
court and says, "Your honor, my client is innocent. First of
all, he did not steal the chickens; secondly, he returned the
chickens; and finally, the chickens were not worth very
much anyway." It sounds as if what I have been saying is:
First of all, it is not a lie; second, if it is a lie it is a permissible
lie; and finally, the truth is not worth knowing in the first
place. Since the truth will do more harm than good, what is
the point of telling the truth?

Nevertheless, in the real world there certainly are
exceptions. First, an exception must be admitted in a situation in which disclosure is necessary in order to secure the
cooperation of the patient in his treatment. Second, there are
situations in which the patient is bound to discover the truth
and he may learn the nature of his illness in circumstances
that will cause greater harm than would result from disclosure by the physician. In some cases, early, sensitive disclosure may constitute the better part of valor.

These exceptions are formulated in a somewhat different manner by Dr. Abraham S. Abraham in *Nishmat Avraham, Yoreh De'ah* 338:3. The author distinguishes between
diagnosis in the early stages of an illness and discovery of a
terminal condition in the final stages of the illness. He
remarks that, in the early stages of the illness, one should
inform the family *and* the patient, both in order to secure the
patient's cooperation and to assuage the patient's fears. Of
course, one must be very supportive and stress the fact that
therapy is available and that there is great hope. However,
when the malady is discovered at an advanced stage and only
palliative treatment is available, Dr. Abraham sees no point

in informing the patient. I can accept that recommendation up to a point. I can conceive of the case, for example, of a very independent middle-aged person to whom the physician has already lied. The patient's tumor was surgically removed and, at the time, there was no reason to disclose the malignancy. Later, the patient develops such symptoms as weight loss, blood in the stool, lack of appetite, and nausea. At this point no cure is available. The physician wishes to administer radiation therapy for palliative purposes, but the patient does not know what is wrong with him. After making a recitation of the symptoms and a review of laboratory reports, the physician informs the patient that he must undergo radiation therapy. The patient may say, "Doctor, why are you worried about my loss of weight? For years you have been telling me to lose weight. Are you concerned about the blood in my stool? I have hemorrhoids, you know that. I don't have any appetite because my wife is not cooking as well as she used to. Occasional nausea—for that you want me to take radiation? Doctor, you know that radiation can cause leukemia! Do you want me to expose myself to that risk just because of a little nausea?" Under those circumstances, the physician will certainly find it necessary to reveal the diagnosis to the patient in order to obtain his cooperation even for palliative treatment. Of course, the physician must be careful not to inform the patient of the severity of his condition and of the fact that the treatment is merely palliative in nature.

Not all patients are alike. There are some clinical symptoms that one cannot mask, disguise, or "misinterpret" if one is treating, for example, a patient who happens to be a physician or a professor of pharmacology. Indeed, in the present-day world, it is difficult to conceal the import of such symptoms from any educated and sophisticated patient. This is even more likely to be the case in the advanced stages of a malady than in early stages. Under these circumstances, one has no choice; one must confirm to the patient what the patient already knows. However, at any stage of illness, the patient should be given unfavorable information only to the extent that it is necessary for his physical and psychic well-being. And, even more significantly, his condition and prognosis should be portrayed in the most favorable light possible under the circumstances.

Simply for purposes of intellectual honesty, let me also cite the statement of Rabbi Judah the Pious, *Sefer Chasidim*, no. 154. Rabbi Judah writes of a physician who is reported to have had the remarkable capability of being able to determine whether or not a patient would die simply by examining his urine. I marvel at this doctor who, without laboratory facilities, was able to examine a specimen of urine and determine that the patient was afflicted with a terminal illness. Be that as it may, Rabbi Judah declares that, under such circumstances, if the patient tells the physician, "Do not hide anything from me. I know you doctors. You do not tell the truth because you are afraid of causing *tiruf ha-da'at*. But I would be happier and more at peace if I knew the truth," the rule is as follows: If the patient does not wish to live and if he is also experiencing excruciating pain, one may tell him the truth. Rabbi Abraham Price, in his commentary on *Sefer Chasidim*, *Nishmat Avraham*, advances what seems to me to be a cogent analysis of the approach outlined there. The exception posited by *Sefer Chasidim*, he states, is limited to a case in which the patient is suffering great pain and, as a result, is already in a state of *tiruf ha-da'at*. Although it is forbidden to hasten the death of any patient, nevertheless— since this patient is already experiencing a type of *tiruf ha-da'at* in that he is already in a state of mental anguish and he truly wishes to die in order to be spared further agony— any information he will receive about his condition will serve only to calm him. It is only in this type of situation, in which *tiruf ha-da'at* is already present, that disclosure does no harm and may do some good. I cannot say that the approach of *Sefer Chasidim* is necessarily normative Jewish law. In instances in which rulings of *Sefer Chasidim* are incorporated in the writings of the early talmudic commentators and codes of Jewish law, they become accepted practice by virtue of that incorporation. In instances such as this, in which *Sefer Chasidim* is not cited by early authorities, its comments are not necessarily to be regarded as normative Halachah.

PRACTICAL APPLICATIONS

What should be done when one is confronted with a patient who is suffering from a serious disease or a patient who is suffering from a terminal illness? Clearly, the concerns that point in the direction of disclosure are cogent. They include the concern that the individual have the opportunity for recitation of *viduy*, or final confession before God, and repentance. He should have the opportunity to put his affairs in order and to make provisions for his family. Those are concerns that were recognized by rabbinic authorities as well. They counsel that the patient be told, "Confess and do not be fearful, for many people have confessed and did not die, and many who did not confess have died. Some people survive in the merit of having repented and confessed." That is the traditional manner in which one recites *viduy* with a terminally ill patient. On several occasions I have taken the liberty of shortening and paraphrasing this statement by telling the patient, "*Viduy* is a *segulah* for longevity; the merit of *viduy* can lead to a long life." Recitation of *viduy* can indeed reverse the heavenly edict and cause a favorable decree to be issued.

Rabbi Abraham Danzig, *Chochmat Adam* 151:10, reports a practice that certainly constitutes an appropriate paradigm. He reports that the practice of the Jewish community of Berlin was that, if a person did not attend synagogue for three consecutive days, officers of the *Bikur Cholim* society would pay a visit to that person at his home. The *Bikur*

Cholim society did not make house calls for every case of sniffles. In eighteenth-century Berlin, a Jew was absent from the synagogue for three consecutive days only if seriously ill; one did not miss communal worship because of mere discomfort. Accordingly, if a person did not appear in the synagogue for three days, it was assumed that he was seriously ill. The *Bikur Cholim* society visited the patient and informed him that they had come to recite *viduy* with him. But the patients did not become afraid because they knew that the society habitually visited everyone who was absent from the synagogue for three days. Many such patients experienced a complete recovery and resumed their normal practice of attending synagogue services three times a day.

It seems to me that this constitutes a model for how the modern-day physician should comport himself. Long before a definitive diagnosis is possible, the physician should be able to say to the patient, "Look, I tell all my patients the same thing: We are going to do laboratory tests. We may even put you in the hospital for observation. I hope that it will turn out to be nothing, but I give every patient the same advice anyway." The physician should then proceed to tell the patient that any medical condition may become serious and that one should order one's affairs accordingly. Most significantly, this information should be conveyed long before the situation is known to be serious. Moreover, the emphasis must be not so much on *what* is said, because in some situations there is no way to avoid the truth, but on *how* it is said. The tone of voice, the facial expression, and the demeanor of the physician are tremendously significant, and even more important than the spoken words.

The physician has absolutely no right whatsoever to tell any patient that there is nothing that can be done for him. He has absolutely no right whatsoever to tell the patient that there is no hope. Even if the nature of the disease has to be identified, and even if the severity of the illness must be spelled out, it should always be in a context and in a manner that is supportive, hopeful, and assuring, and that conveys the message that everything that can be done on behalf of the patient will be done.

I am well aware of the fact that there is great resistance to the policy that I have outlined. But since the teachings and values of Judaism are often unpopular, that is not surprising. I will conclude with a brief story. Years ago, when I was a young student, I remember someone returning to the yeshiva after having spent a *Shabbat* in Lakewood, New Jersey. Rabbi Aaron Kotler, of blessed memory, used to deliver his weekly *shi'ur* on Saturday evening after the conclusion of the Sabbath. Lakewood at the time was a popular resort area, and many Jews went there for weekends. Many visitors would go to the yeshiva there on Saturday evenings to hear Rabbi Kotler's discourse, and occasionally one would ask a question during the course of the *shi'ur*. The story that was brought back was that on the previous Saturday evening, a gentleman had interrupted Rabbi Kotler and asked him a question. Rabbi Kotler answered. The man proceeded to argue with Rabbi Kotler. Rabbi Kotler answered a second time. The man continued to argue until finally Rabbi Kotler exclaimed, "If you disagree with me, it must be a sign that I am right because the views of *ba'alei battim* are opposite to the views of Torah. So it is written in the *Sema, Choshen Mishpat* 3:23." The actual comment of *Sema* is not quite as strong as the words quoted in his name. However, *Sema*—citing a responsum of Maharil—does state that what is accepted as normative by the general public and what is regarded as normative by Torah scholars are unfortunately, more often than not, not one and the same. Often they are diametrically opposed. Moral dilemmas should not be resolved on the basis of intuition. *Vox populi* is not always intuitively reflective of *vox Dei* and it is to the latter that our ears must be attuned.

4

COMMUNICABLE DISEASES AND THE PHYSICIAN'S OBLIGATION TO HEAL

Fred Rosner, M.D.

It is axiomatic in Judaism that human life is of infinite value and that all efforts must be applied to heal the sick, to cure illness, and to prolong life. Even the Sabbath and Yom Kippur must be desecrated if necessary to save a human life, and all biblical and rabbinic rules and regulations except the cardinal three must be suspended in the face of danger to life. These three exceptions are idolatry, murder, and forbidden sexual relationships such as incest. A person with only a few moments to live has the same rights and is considered just as valuable in the eyes of God as a person with many years of life ahead.

Judaism never condones the deliberate destruction of human life except in judicial execution for certain criminal acts, in self-defense, or in time of war. One also may not sacrifice one life to save another life or even many other lives. Many of the principles of Jewish medical ethics are based on this concept of the infinite value of human life. He who saves one life, asserts the Talmud (*Sanhedrin* 37a), is as if he saved a whole world. Even a few moments of life are worthwhile. Judaism is a "right to life" religion. The obligation to save lives is both an individual and a communal obligation. A physician is divinely licensed and biblically mandated to use his medical skills to heal the sick and thereby prolong and preserve life.

How far does the physician's obligation to heal extend? Is the physician obligated to endanger his own life to treat patients with contagious and/or communicable diseases? How much risk to his own health and life is the physician allowed or obligated to undertake in the care of his patients? Does the general obligation on all Jews of visiting the sick (*bikur cholim*) also include visits to patients with contagious diseases? These questions are the subject of this chapter.

THE PHYSICIAN'S LICENSE
AND OBLIGATION TO HEAL

The ethical and legal question of whether or not a person is allowed in Jewish law to become a physician and heal the sick is based on the biblical statement in which the Lord asserts: "I will put none of the diseases upon you that I put upon the Egyptians for I am the Lord that heals you" (Exodus 15:26).

The final phrase, "I am the Lord that heals you," literally translated from the Hebrew means "I am the Lord your physician." The Karaites interpreted this scriptural phrase literally and totally rejected the permissibility of human healing. They vehemently objected to medicine and physicians and relied totally on prayer for their healing, as stated in the Talmud: Man must always pray not to become ill, for if he becomes so, it is demanded of him to show merit in order to be healed (*Shabbat* 32a). Rabbi Abraham Ibn Ezra states that just as God healed the undrinkable waters at Marah for the Jews, so too God will remove all plagues from the face of the earth and there will be no need for physicians.

Elsewhere, the Talmud (*Sanhedrin* 101a), asks: If we are told that God "will put none of the diseases upon you," what need is there for a cure? Rabbi Yochanan answers that the meaning of the verse is as follows: If you will hearken [to the voice of the Lord], I will not bring disease upon you, but if you will not, I will; yet even so, "I am the Lord that heals you." Rabbi Baruch Halevi Epstein, in his commentary known as Torah Temimah, explains that the intent of the scriptural phrase is to show that the illness of the Egyptians was incurable, as it is written: "The boil of Egypt . . . wherefrom one cannot be healed" (Deuteronomy 28:27). However, afflictions of the Israelites can be healed by God.

In his biblical commentary, Rashi explains "I am the Lord that heals you" to mean that God teaches the laws of the Torah in order to save man from disease. Rashi uses the analogy of a physician who tells his patient not to eat a particular food lest it bring him into danger from disease. So too, continues Rashi, obedience to God's commandments is "health to your body and marrow to your bones" (Proverbs 3:8). In a similar vein, the extratalmudic collection of biblical interpretation known as the *Mechilta* asserts that the words of Torah are life as well as health: "They are life unto those that found them and health to all their flesh" (Proverbs 4:22). Other commentators, including Sifsei Chachamim and Rabbi Samson Raphael Hirsch, extend this thought by propounding that the Divine Law restores health and certainly prevents illness from occurring, thus serving as preventive medicine against all physical and social evil.

Rabbi Jacob ben Asher, known as Ba'al Haturim, states that heavenly cure comes easily, whereas manmade cures come with difficulty. Rabbi Meir Leib ben Yechiel Michael, known as Malbim, interprets the phrase "I am the Lord that heals you" to include mental or spiritual illness and to imply that God's statutes are for our benefit, not His.

The multitude of interpretations of the scriptural verse "I am the Lord that heals you" indicates that this phrase is not to be taken literally. There is no absolute prohibition inherent in this verse against becoming a physician and healing the sick. In fact, specific permission, sanction, and even mandate for the physician to practice medicine is given in the Torah based on the rabbinic interpretation of the biblical phrase "and heal he shall heal" (Exodus 21:19). This phrase relates to compensation for personal injuries, such compensation consisting of five items: payment for the physical damage or injury, payment for loss of time from work, payment for pain, payment for shame incurred, and payment of the physician's fees and medical bills. The Sages in the Talmud interpret the duplicate mention of healing in the phrase "heal he shall heal" to mean that authorization was granted by God to a physician to heal (*Baba Kamma* 85a). The Bible implies that it is as if there are two physicians: One is Almighty God, the true Healer of the sick; and the other is the human physician, who serves as an instrument of God or an extension of Him in ministering to the sick.

Many biblical commentators, including Hirsch and Torah Temimah, echo this talmudic teaching. By the insistence or emphasis expressed in the double wording, the Bible opposes the erroneous idea espoused by the Karaites that recourse to medicine shows lack of trust and faith in divine assistance. The Bible takes it for granted that medical therapy is used, and actually requires it. The Mechilta and Malbim explain "heal he shall heal" to mean that the patient must be repeatedly healed if the illness or injury recurs or is exacerbated. Ibn Ezra seems to limit the physician's license to heal in that he permits only external or "manmade" wounds to be healed by physicians; internal wounds or ailments should, in his view, be left to God. Ibn Ezra's restrictive view is rejected by most codes of Jewish law, including Rabbi Joseph Karo's *Shulchan Aruch.*[1]

Moses Maimonides derives the biblical sanction for a physician to heal from the scriptural commandment "And thou shalt restore it to him" (Deuteronomy 22:2), which refers to the restoration of lost property. In his Mishnah commentary, Maimonides asserts:

> It is obligatory from the Torah for the physician to heal the sick and this is included in the explanation of the scriptural phrase "And thou shalt restore it to him," meaning to heal his body. If he sees him in danger and is able to save him, he should save him with his body or his money or his wisdom.[2]

Thus, Maimonides states that the law of the restoration of a lost object also includes the restoration of the health of one's fellow human being. If a person has "lost his health" and the physician is able to restore it, he is obligated to do so. In two separate places in his biblical commentary (Exodus 21:19 and Deuteronomy 22:2), Torah Temimah asks why Maimonides fails to invoke the phrase "heal he shall heal" as a warrant for the physician to heal. He answers that this phrase from Exodus only *grants permission* for a physician to heal, whereas the phrase in Deuteronomy, "And thou shalt restore it to him," makes it *obligatory* upon the physician to heal.

The Mishnah commentator Rabbi Obadiah of Bertinoro[3] also states that it is obligatory for a physician to heal his fellow humans because the precept of restoring a lost object includes the restoration of lost health, and thus it is a commandment (*mitzvah*) to do so even if the patient had sworn not to derive any benefit from that physician.

---

1. *Orach Chayim* 328:3.
2. M. Maimonides, *Mishnah Commentary* on *Nedarim* 4:4.
3. O. Bertinoro, *Mishnah Commentary* on *Nedarim* 4:4.

Maimonides' reasoning is probably based upon a key passage in the Talmud: "Whence do we know that one must save his neighbor from the loss of himself? From the verse 'and thou shalt restore it to him'" (*Sanhedrin* 73a). Thus even if a person is attempting suicide or refuses treatment for illness, one is obligated to intervene to save that person's life and health.

The second scriptural mandate for a physician to heal is based on the phrase "Do not stand idly by the blood of your neighbor" (Leviticus 19:16). This passage refers to the duties of human beings to their fellow humans. One example cited in the Talmud is the following: "Whence do we know that if a man sees his neighbor drowning or mauled by beasts or attacked by robbers, he is bound to save him? From the verse 'Do not stand idly by the blood of your neighbor'" (*Sanhedrin* 73a).

Maimonides codifies this talmudic passage in his *Mishneh Torah* as follows:

> Whoever is able to save another and does not save him trangresses the commandment "Do not stand idly by the blood of your neighbor." Similarly, if one sees another drowning in the sea, or being attacked by bandits, or being attacked by a wild animal, and is able to rescue him . . . and does not rescue him . . . he transgresses the injunction "Do not stand idly by the blood of your neighbor."[4]

A case of drowning or of attack is considered as the potential loss of the entire body, and one is obligated to save it. Certainly one must cure even a disease that afflicts only part of the body.

In summary, it is evident in Jewish tradition that divine license is given to a physician to heal based on the interpretation of the biblical phrase "Heal he shall heal." Many

---

4. M. Maimonides, *Mishneh Torah, Hilchot Rotze'ach* 1:14.

Jewish scholars, such as Maimonides and Bertinoro, claim that healing the sick is not only allowed but is obligatory. Karo's *Shulchan Aruch* seems to combine both thoughts: "The Torah gave permission to the physician to heal; moreover, it is a religious precept and is included in the category of saving life; and if he withholds his services, it is considered as shedding blood."[5]

THE PATIENT'S OBLIGATION
TO SEEK HEALING

It is clear from our discussion thus far that a physician is divinely licensed and biblically obligated to heal the sick because of the Jewish concept of the supreme value of human life. Is a patient authorized, however, or perhaps mandated, to seek healing from a physician? Is a patient who asks a physician to heal him denying Divine Providence? Is illness an affliction from God that serves as punishment for wrongdoing? Does a patient forego atonement for his sin by not accepting the suffering imposed by Divine Judgment, and instead seeking medical care? Is there a distinction between heavenly afflictions and human-induced illness or injury?

The Talmud states that upon going to be phlebotomized, one should recite the following prayer: "May it be Your will, O Lord, my God, that this operation may be a cure for me, and may You heal me, for You are a faithful healing God, and Your healing is sure, since men have no power to heal but this is a habit with them" (*Berachot* 60a).

The Talmud describes a patient going to a physician for an operative procedure, thus indicating that it is permissible for the patient to do so provided he recognizes that God is the true healer and that the physician is acting as an agent of

---

5. J. Karo, *Shulchan Aruch, Yoreh De'ah* 336.

the Divine Healer. On the other hand, the talmudic statement continues with an assertion by Abaye that a patient
should not utter such a prayer because the Torah gives
specific sanction for human healing in the phrase "Heal he
shall heal." Therefore, says Abaye, a patient *should* seek the
help of a physician. A similar but not identical prayer is
found in Maimonides' *Mishneh Torah*[6] and Karo's *Shulchan
Aruch*.[7]

Moses Nachmanides offers a rather negative attitude
toward the question of the patient seeking medical aid, in his
commentary on the scriptural phrase "And My soul shall not
abhor you" (Leviticus 26:11). "During the era of the prophets," said Nachmanides, himself a physician, "the righteous,
even when ill, did not seek out physicians, only prophets."
What, therefore, is the need for physicians? The physician's
purpose is to advise on which foods and beverages to avoid
in order to prevent illness, in Nachmanides' view. He
explains the phrase "Heal he shall heal" to mean that the
physician is allowed to practice medicine; however, the
patient may not seek the physician's healing but should turn
to Divine Providence. Nachmanides states that only people
who do not believe in the healing powers of God turn to
physicians for their cure, and that for such individuals the
Torah sanctions the physician to heal.

Other than the Karaites, who strongly objected to
physicians and medicines, Nachmanides seems to stand
alone in his apparent prohibition of the seeking of medical
aid. Perhaps he refers only to the righteous who are free of
illness because of their piety and who thus do not require
human healing. Perhaps the general populace, however,
even devout believers in God, are allowed to seek human
healing. Such an interpretation of Nachmanides' discussion
is offered by Rabbi David ben Shmuel Halevi, known as Taz

---

6. M. Maimonides, *Mishneh Torah, Hilchot Berachot* 10:21.
7. J. Karo, *Shulchan Aruch, Orach Chayim* 230:4.

or Turei Zahav, in his commentary on Karo's code.[8] It may also be that Nachmanides agrees with Ibn Ezra, who states that human-induced illnesses may be healed, and only in the case of divine afflictions and illnesses is the patient prohibited from seeking human healing.

The strongest evidence in Jewish sources that a patient is permitted to seek healing from a physician is found in Maimonides' *Mishneh Torah* as follows:

> A person should set his heart that his body be healthy and strong in order that his soul be upright to know the Lord. For it is impossible for man to understand and comprehend the wisdoms [of the world] if he is hungry and ailing or if one of his limbs is aching. . . .[9]

He also recommends,[10] as does the Talmud (*Sanhedrin* 17b), that no wise person should reside in a city that does not have a physician. Maimonides' position is further expanded and codified as follows:

> Since when the body is healthy and sound [one treads] in the ways of the Lord, it being impossible to understand or know anything of the knowledge of the Creator when one is sick, it is obligatory upon man to avoid things which are detrimental to the body and to acclimate himself to things which heal and fortify it.[11]

Numerous talmudic citations indicate that patients are allowed and even required to seek medical attention. Thus it is said that one who is in pain should go to a physician (*Baba Kamma* 46b); that if one is bitten by a snake, a physician is

---

8. Taz's commentary on J. Karo's *Shulchan Aruch, Yoreh De'ah* 336:1.
9. M. Maimonides, *Mishneh Torah, Hilchot Deot* 3:3.
10. Ibid., 4:23.
11. Ibid., 4:1.

called even on the Sabbath because all restrictions are set aside in the event of possible danger to human life (*Yoma* 83b). If one's eye is afflicted, one may prepare and apply medication even on the Sabbath (*Abodah Zarah* 28b). Rabbi Judah the Prince, compiler of the Mishnah, suffered from an eye ailment and consulted his physician, Mar Samuel, who cured the ailment by placing a vial of chemicals under the rabbi's pillow so that the powerful vapors would penetrate the eye (*Baba Metzia* 85b). In the case of bodily injury, if the offender tells the victim that he will bring a physician who will heal for no fee, the victim can object and say, "A physician who heals for nothing is worth nothing" (*Baba Kamma* 85a).

From these and other talmudic passages, it is evident that an individual is not only allowed but probably required to seek medical attention when he is ill. Further evidence to support this contention is the biblical precept requiring the construction of parapets around roofs for the prevention of accidents (Deuteronomy 22:8). From this precept we see that humans should not rely on miracles or Divine Providence alone but must avail themselves of whatever they can to maintain life and health, including recourse to physicians. One might arrive at the same conclusion if one were to interpret literally the biblical admonition "Take therefore good heed unto yourselves" (Deuteronomy 4:15). Thus it is clear that people are obligated to care for their health and life. They are charged with preserving them. They must eat and drink and sustain themselves and must seek healing when they are ill in order to be able to serve the Lord in a state of good health.

THE PHYSICIAN'S OBLIGATION TO HEAL PATIENTS WITH CONTAGIOUS DISEASES

Having established the physician's divine mandate to heal the sick, one can ask: How far does this mandate extend? Is a physician obligated to treat a patient with a contagious disease if there is a risk that he might contract the illness from the patient? Is a physician obligated to endanger his own health or life to restore the health or save the life of a patient?

We have already mentioned that Jewish law requires that if one sees one's neighbor drowning or being mauled by beasts or attacked by robbers, he is bound to save him (*Sanhedrin* 73a). This rule is codified by Maimonides[12] and Karo.[13] Elsewhere, Karo[14] rules that if one observes a ship sinking with people on board, or a river flooding over its banks, thereby endangering lives, or a pursued person whose life is in danger, one is obligated to desecrate the Sabbath to save the victims. The commentaries of Rabbi Israel Meir Kagan, known as *Mishnah Berurah*,[15] and of Rabbi Abraham Zvi Hirsch Eisenstadt, known as *Pitchei Teshuvah*,[16] add that if there is mortal danger involved to the rescuer, he is not obligated to endanger his life because his life takes precedence over that of his fellow man. If there is only a small risk (*sofek sakanah*) to the rescuer, he should carefully evaluate the potential danger and act accordingly.

How should a physician proceed if the patient is suffering from a contagious disease? Is the physician allowed to refuse to treat the patient because of the risk or because of his fear of contracting the disease? What if the risk is very small, or *sofek sakanah*? What is the definition of *sofek sakanah*? If

---

12. M. Maimonides, *Mishneh Torah, Hilchot Rotze'ach* 1:14.
13. J. Karo, *Shulchan Aruch, Choshen Mishpat* 426:1.
14. J. Karo, *Shulchan Aruch, Orach Chayim* 329:8.
15. I. M. Kagan, *Mishnah Berurah* 329:19.
16. A. Z. H. Eisenstadt, *Pitchei Teshuvah, Choshen Mishpat* 426:2.

there is a 50 percent chance of the physician's contracting the disease from the patient, Halachah would certainly agree that such odds are more than *sofek sakanah* and that the physician would not be obligated to care for that patient without taking precautionary measures to protect himself. If he wishes to care for the patient in spite of the risk, his act is considered to be a pious one (*midat chasidut*) by some writers and folly (*chasid shoteh*) by others. If the risk is very remote, however, the physician must care for the patient because "the Lord preserveth the simpletons" (Psalm 116:6). This phrase is invoked in the Talmud (*Yebamot* 12b) in relation to the remote danger of conception in a minor child and discussed in great detail by Rabbi Moshe Feinstein[17] in a lengthy responsum concerning the use of a contraceptive device by a woman for whom pregnancy would be life-threatening. Contraception, states Feinstein, is permissible for *sofek sakanah* but not if the risk is extremely small. Rabbi Shneur Zalman of Lublin[18] and Rabbi Chayim Ozer Grodzensky,[19] respectively, discuss whether the foregoing biblical phrase is invoked for a minor risk (less than 50 percent) or for a very remote and rare risk.

Rabbi Yitzchak Zilberstein[20] discusses the case of a female physician in her first trimester of pregnancy who is called to see a seriously ill patient with rubella (German measles). The physician is at 50 percent risk of acquiring rubella and possibly giving birth to a baby with serious birth defects (blindness, deafness, or mental retardation), or she might have an abortion or a stillbirth. Although there are no fetal indications in Halachah that would allow abortion, Zilberstein posits that Halachah considers miscarriage to be a situation of *pikuach nefesh* (danger to life) and therefore rules

---

17. M. Feinstein, *Responsa Iggrot Moshe, Even Haezer*, no. 63.
18. S. Zalman, *Responsa Torat Chesed, Even Haezer*, no. 44.
19. C. O. Grodzensky, *Responsa Achiezer*, part 1, no. 23.
20. Y. Zilberstein, *Assia* (Jerusalem), vol. 11 (1986), pp. 5–11.

that the pregnant physician is not obligated to care for the patient with rubella.

The question as to whether or not a person is obligated or allowed to subject himself to risk in order to save another's life is discussed in great detail in several recent articles.[21-24] This question is related to the well-known difference of opinion recorded in the Talmuds. The Jerusalem Talmud[25] posits that a person is obligated to potentially endanger his life if the risk is small (*sofek sakanah*) to save the life of a fellow human being from certain danger (*vadai sakanah*, or great risk). This position is supported by Rabbi Meir Hacohen, known as *Hagohat Maimuni*, as cited by Karo,[26] and by Karo himself in his *Bet Yoseph* commentary.[27] On the other hand, the Babylonian Talmud[28] voices the opinion that one is not obligated to endanger one's life even if the risk is small to save that of another. The ruling from the Jerusalem Talmud is omitted from the Codes of Alfasi (Rif), Maimonides, Asher ben Yehiel (Rosh), Jacob ben Asher (Tur), and Isserles (Rema), suggesting that Halachah rejects that position.

The prevailing opinion among the various rabbinic sources seems to be the one cited by Rabbi David Ibn Zimra, known as Radvaz.[29] If there is great danger to the rescuer, he

---

21. M. Hershler, *Halachah Urefuah*, vol. 2 (Jerusalem: Regensburg Institute, 1981), pp. 52–57.

22. M. Y. Sloshitz, *Halachah Urefuah*, vol. 3 (Jerusalem: Regensburg Institute, 1983), pp. 158–163.

23. A. Metzger, *Harefuah Le'or HaHalachah*, vol. 4 (Jerusalem, 1985), pp. 10–34.

24. A. S. Abraham, *Hamayan* (Jerusalem, 1982), pp. 31ff.

25. Terumot, end of chap. 8, according to *Ha'amek She'elah, She'iltot* 147:1.

26. J. Karo, *Keseph Mishneh*, commentary on *Hilchot Rotze'ach* 1:14.

27. J. Karo, *Bet Yoseph, Tur Shulchan Aruch, Choshen Mishpat* 426.

28. *Sanhedrin* 73a, according to *Agudat Aizov, Derushim* folio 3b and *Hashmatot* folio 38b.

29. D. Zimra, *Responsa Radvaz*, part 5 (part 2 in *Leshonot HaRambam*, section 1, 582); *Responsa Radvaz* 3:627; and *She'iltot Radvaz* 1:52.

is not allowed to attempt to save his fellow man; if he nevertheless does so, he is called a pious fool. If the danger to the rescuer is small and the danger to his fellow man very great, the rescuer is allowed but not obligated to attempt the rescue, and if he does so his act is called an act of loving kindness (*midat chasidut*). If there is no risk at all to the rescuer or if the risk is very small or remote, he is obligated to try to save his fellow man. If he refuses to do so, he is guilty of transgressing the commandment "Thou shalt not stand idly by the blood of thy fellow man" (Leviticus 19:16). This approach is also adopted by recent rabbinic decisors, including Rabbi Moshe Feinstein[30] and Rabbi Eliezer Yehudah Waldenberg.[31] If the risk to physicians and other healthcare personnel in caring for patients with contagious diseases such as tuberculosis, or communicable diseases such as AIDS, is very small, a physician is obligated under Jewish law to care for such patients. The risk of contracting AIDS from the prick of a needle that has been in contact with AIDS-infected blood is less than a fraction of 1 percent.

The same logic is applied to allow, but not require, healthy people to donate a kidney to save the life of a close relative dying of kidney failure. Most rabbis—including Rabbi Immanuel Jakobovits,[32] Rabbi Ovadiah Yosef,[33] Rabbi Jacob Joseph Weiss,[34] Rabbi Eliezer Waldenberg,[35] Rabbi Moshe Meiselman,[36] and Rabbi Moshe Hershler[37]—support this halachic position. A person who donates a kidney to save a life is considered to have performed a *midat chasidut* because the donor accepts the very small risk inherent in the

---

30. M. Feinstein, *Responsa Iggrot Moshe, Yoreh De'ah* 2:174, p. 4.

31. E. Y. Waldenberg, *Responsa Tzitz Eliezer*, vol. 10, p. 7.

32. I. Jakobovits, personal communication, August 1968.

33. O. Yosef, *Halachah Urefuah*, vol. 3 (1983), pp. 61–63.

34. J. J. Weiss, Responsa *Minchat Yitzchok*, part 6, no. 103, p. 2.

35. E. Y. Waldenberg, Responsa *Tzitz Eliezer*, vol. 10, no. 25, p. 7.

36. M. Meiselman, *Halachah Urefuah*, vol. 2 (1981), pp. 114–121.

37. M. Hershler, *Halachah Urefuah*, vol. 2 (1981), pp. 122–127.

induction of anesthesia, the risk and discomfort of the surgery required to remove his healthy kidney, and the risk to his own health of being left with only one kidney. Organ transplantation in Jewish law is discussed in greater detail elsewhere.[38]

VISITING PATIENTS WITH INFECTIOUS DISEASES

Judaism views visiting the sick as more than a social obligation—it is a commandment. In Jewish tradition the visit itself entails more than paying a social call. Because there were no hospitals in biblical and talmudic times, a person who visited a sick friend or relative was expected to provide for the physical as well as the emotional needs of the patient.

In addition to cheering up the patient and giving him the courage to recover, the visitor would help him by performing necessary tasks such as cooking or housecleaning. Jewish law also requires that the visitor pray for the patient's recovery. These three activities are all essential components of *bikur cholim*—visiting the sick—and are applicable to this very day.

The reason that every Jew is required to visit the sick is that God visits the sick and we must emulate Him. This general rule is based on the verse "You shall walk after the Lord your God" (Deuteronomy 13:5). Since the literal command is clearly impossible to fulfill, the reference is to our obligation to try to emulate His attributes. God also sets eternal examples for us to follow by blessing bridegrooms, adorning brides, burying the dead, and comforting mourn-

---

38. F. Rosner, *Modern Medicine and Jewish Ethics* (Hoboken, NJ, and New York: Ktav and Yeshiva University Press, 1986), pp. 255–275; and in chapters 9 and 10 of this book.

ers (Genesis *Rabbah* 8:13). Just as He visited the sick, so, too, should we (*Sotah* 14a). He visited the patriarch Abraham when he was recovering from his circumcision, as it is written, "And the Lord appeared unto him" (Genesis 18:1). Another passage, "You shall show them the way they must walk (Exodus 18:20), also refers to the duty of visiting the sick (*Baba Kamma* 100a and *Baba Metzia* 30b).

By tending the needs of a sick patient, one may help not only to restore health but also to save a life, as illustrated in the Talmud (*Nedarim* 40a) in an incident in which Rabbi Akiba visited and cared for one of his disciples, who was ill. The disciple said, "My master, you have revived me." In addition to dealing directly with the patient's physical and emotional needs, a visitor should pray in the patient's behalf. "There is no limit to the visiting of the sick" (*Nedarim* 39b) has multiple interpretations. One sage states that it means the reward has no limit. Another explains that it means the obligation applies to everyone, without limit: even a person of prominence must visit a simple man. Yet another states that it means there is no limit to the frequency of such visits, even if they number a hundred a day.

Many other rules and recommendations are associated with visiting the sick. For example, some hours are preferable to others for *bikur cholim*. As discussed on page 39, one should abstain from visiting a patient during the first three hours and the last three hours of the day, lest one misjudge the patient's status and not pray for him or care for him properly.

Moreover, one should not visit patients who are suffering from abdominal distress, eye diseases, or headaches—the first because the patient may be embarrassed, and the latter two because speech may be harmful to him (*Nedarim* 41a). In addition, one should not visit a patient until his fever has subsided. Close relatives and friends usually visit first, and more distant relatives and acquaintances visit only after three days. If the illness occurred suddenly, all may visit simultaneously (*Yerushalmi Pe'ah* 3:17).

Does the obligation to visit the sick extend to visiting patients with contagious diseases, such as tuberculosis, hepatitis, or pneumonia? The Torah tells us not to intentionally place ourselves in danger: "Take heed to thyself, and take care of thy life" (Deuteronomy 4:19); "Take good care of your lives" (Deuteronomy 4:15). The advisability of avoiding danger is repeated throughout the Bible, the Talmud, and codes of Jewish law in the positive commandment of making a parapet for one's roof so that no man may fall therefrom (Deuteronomy 22:8). Moses Maimonides enumerates a variety of prohibitions, all based upon the consideration of the potential of being harmful to life. They are quoted verbatim since they so eloquently illustrate the point under discussion:

> It makes no difference whether it be one's roof or anything else that is dangerous and might possibly be a stumbling block to someone and cause his death—for example, if one has a well or a pit, with or without water, in his yard—the owner is obligated to build an enclosing wall ten handbreadths high, or else to put a cover over it lest someone fall into it and be killed. Similarly, regarding any obstacle which is dangerous to life, there is a positive commandment to remove it and to beware of it, and to be particularly careful in this matter. . . .
>
> Many things are forbidden by the Sages because they are dangerous to life. If one disregards any of these and says, "If I want to put myself in danger, what concern is it to others?" or "I am not particular about such things," disciplinary flogging is inflicted upon him.
>
> The following are the acts prohibited: One may not put his mouth to a flowing pipe of water and drink from it, or drink at night from rivers or ponds, lest he swallow a leech while unable to see. Nor may one drink water that has been left uncovered, lest he drink it after a snake or other poisonous reptile has drunk from it, and die. . . .

One should not put small change or *denar* into his mouth lest they carry the dried saliva of one who suffers from an infectious skin disease or leprosy, or lest they carry perspiration, since all human perspiration is poisonous except that coming from the face.

Similarly, one should not put the palm of his hand under his arm, for his hand might possibly have touched a leper or some harmful substance, since the hands are constantly in motion. Nor should one put a dish of food under his seat even during a meal, lest something harmful fall into it without his noticing it.

Similarly, one should not stick a knife into a citron or a radish lest someone fall on the point and be killed. Similarly, one should not walk near a leaning wall or over a shaking bridge or enter a ruin or pass through any other such dangerous place.[39]

This quotation from Maimonides certainly emphasizes the point that placing one's health or life at risk is absolutely prohibited. Similar prohibitions against endangering one's life are found in most later codes of Jewish law, including Karo's *Shulchan Aruch*. The latter devotes an entire chapter to "the positive commandment of removing any object or obstacle which constitutes a danger to life."[40] Elsewhere, Karo reiterates the prohibitions against drinking water left uncovered, putting money in one's mouth, putting one's hand or a loaf of bread under the armpit, leaving a knife in a fruit, consuming unappetizing food, and using dirty pots or dishes.[41] He further states that two people should not drink from the same cup[42] and that one should pause between eating fish and meat.[43]

39. M. Maimonides, *Mishneh Torah, Hilchot Rotze'ach* 11:4ff.
40. J. Karo, *Shulchan Aruch, Choshen Mishpat* 427.
41. Ibid., *Yoreh De'ah* 116.
42. Ibid., *Orach Chayim* 170:16.
43. Ibid., 73:2.

Rabbi Moses Isserles, known as Rema, in his gloss on Karo's code, concludes as follows:

> One should avoid all things that might lead to danger because a danger to life is stricter than a prohibition. One should be more concerned about a possible danger to life than a possible prohibition. Therefore, the sages prohibited one from walking in a place of danger, such as near a leaning wall [for fear of collapse], or alone at night [for fear of robbers]. They also prohibited drinking water from rivers at night . . . because [all] these things may lead to danger . . . and he who is concerned with his health [literally: watches his soul] avoids them. And it is prohibited to rely on a miracle or to put one's life in danger by any of the aforementioned or the like.[44]

With this background, the question can be asked again: Does the obligation of visiting the sick include exposing oneself to patients with contagious diseases? Rabbi Jakobovits[45] points out that the question was answered with a qualified affirmation by Isserles in his responsa.[46] Later authorities questioned the need to expose oneself to the hazard of contagion in the fulfillment of the precept of *bikur cholim*. Isserles contends that there is no distinction with regard to visiting the sick between ordinary and infectious diseases, with the sole exception of leprosy.

The nearly universal recommendation for those threatened by plague is flight: "He that remains in the city shall die . . . by the pestilence, but he that goes out . . . he shall live" (Jeremiah 21:9–10). The Talmud states that if you find yourself in a pestilence-ridden town, you are to "gather your feet" (*Baba Kamma* 60b), which means to flee, or to withdraw to a safe place. During an epidemic of plague,

---

44. M. Isserles, *Shulchan Aruch, Yoreh De'ah* 116:5.
45. I. Jakobovits, *Journal of a Rabbi* (New York: Living Books, 1966), p. 157.
46. M. Isserles, *Responsa Ramah*, end of no. 19.

Raba used to close his window shutters (*Baba Kamma* 60b)
because, as Jeremiah (9:20) lamented: "Death is come up
unto our windows." Isserles himself rules that it is proper to
flee from a town in which the plague has broken out.[47]
Others who recommend flight from the plague include
Rabbi Jacob Molin,[48] Rabbi Solomon Luria,[49] Rabbi Isaiah
Horowitz,[50] and many more.[51] Horowitz also cites the
remedy of flight to avoid contracting smallpox, and ex-
presses amazement that "parents are not careful enough to
take away their little ones from the town during the outbreak
of smallpox, called in German *Blattern*."[52] J. David Eisenstein states the following:

> One does not visit patients with *raatan* or lepers or patients
> with contagious diseases and one should not place oneself in
> danger. It is also customary not to visit patients with the
> plague except special individuals engaged for that purpose. In
> the book *Midrash Talpiyot* it is written that he who visits
> patients with the plague should not sit but stand and walk to
> and fro until he leaves. In this manner, the angel of death has
> no authority to control him and to infect him.[53]

According to Isserles, however, one is obligated to visit
patients who have any contagious disease except leprosy.
One examination of this question, according to Jakobovits,[54]

---

47. M. Isserles, *Shulchan Aruch, Yoreh De'ah* 116:5.

48. J. Molin, *Responsa Maharil*, no. 35.

49. S. Luria, *Yam shel shlomo* commentary on *Baba Kamma* 6:26.

50. I. Horowitz, cited by I. Jakobovits in *Jewish Medical Ethics* (New York: Bloch, 1959), p. 12.

51. H. J. Zimmels, *Magicians, Theologians and Doctors* (London: Goldston & Son, 1952), pp. 99–106.

52. Ibid., p. 107.

53. J. D. Eisenstein, *Otzar Dinim Uminhagim* (New York: Hebrew Publishing Co., 1938), p. 49.

54. *Journal of a Rabbi*, p. 156.

based on several talmudic narratives,[55] leads to the conclusion that the ruling of Isserles applies only to an infection that would not endanger the life of the visitor even if he caught it, but that one is not required to risk one's life for the sake of fulfilling merely the rabbinic precept of visiting the sick, nor can anyone be compelled to serve such patients. Elsewhere, Jakobovits[56] asserts that in practice, the view of Isserles did not prevail, and approval was expressed for the custom not to assign visitation of plague-stricken patients to anyone except specially appointed persons who were well paid for their perilous work. Jakobovits also cites the seventeenth-century records of the Portuguese Congregation in Hamburg,[57] which indicate that even the communal physicians and nurses were exempt from the obligation to attend to infectious patients and that the required services were rendered by volunteers entitled to special remuneration.

Rabbi Yekuthiel Yehudah Greenwald, in his famous *Kol Bo al Avelut*,[58] states that if there is hope that the patient will be cured of his illness, one is obligated to visit and serve him even if there is a risk of contracting the disease because, according to the Jerusalem Talmud, as discussed earlier, one is obligated to accept a small risk in order to save one's fellow humans from a definite danger. If there is no chance of saving the patient, however, one should not endanger one's own life by visiting the patient.[59]

The Talmud (*Pesachim* 8b) states that those sent to perform a religious duty do not suffer harm (*shiluchey mitzvah aynon nizakin*). This rule is also codified in Jewish

---

55. *Nedarim* 39b, *Berachot* 22b, and Rashi in *Shabbat* 30a.
56. *Jewish Medical Ethics*, pp. 108–109.
57. J. Cassuto, *Jahrbuch der Juedisch-Literarischen Gesellschaft*, vol. 10 (1912), pp. 252, 280 (in Minutes dated 1664 and 1666).
58. New York and Jerusalem: Feldheim, 1952, p. 17.
59. M. Maimonides, *Mishneh Torah, Hilchot Shemirat Hanefesh* 1:7.

law[60] but only where there is no danger involved to the
person performing the precept. Where there is danger
(*hezekey matzui*), the rule may not apply, and one might be
foolhardy to risk one's life to perform the precept (*chasid
shoteh*). However, if the risk is infinitesimally small (such as
one in a thousand or less), one should fulfill the precept.

In the specific case of AIDS, the risk of contracting the
disease by visiting or touching the patient is nil. No case of
AIDS has yet been reported to have been contracted through
casual contact with an AIDS patient. The virus is transmitted
only through the blood and by sexual contact. Hence,
physicians are obligated to care for patients with AIDS, and
all are obligated to visit patients who have the disease. The
only precaution one need take is to avoid puncturing one's
skin with a needle used to draw blood from or given in an
injection to an AIDS patient. The risk of contracting hepatitis, pneumonia, tuberculosis, or other contagious illnesses
from a patient is usually very small and must be assessed
according to the individual circumstances of the case. Therefore, most patients can be visited and comforted in order to
fulfill the precept of *bikur cholim*. The only exceptions are in
the case of a highly contagious illness or an epidemic.

CONCLUSIONS

According to the precepts of Judaism, every human life is
infinitely valuable. Therefore, physicians and other healthcare providers are obligated to endeavor to heal the sick and
prolong life. Physicians are not only given divine license to
practice medicine; they are also mandated to use their skills
to heal the sick. Failure or refusal to do so, to the resultant

---

60. D. Halevy, Commentary *Turei Zahav* (Taz) on J. Karo's *Shulchan Aruch*,
Orach Chayim 455:3.

detriment of the patient, constitutes a transgression on the part of the physician.

In addition, all people are duty-bound to seek healing from a physician when they are ill and not to rely on divine intervention or faith-healing. They are charged with preserving their health, or restoring it when ill, in order to be fully able to serve the Lord.

The physician's obligation to heal extends even to the care of patients with contagious or communicable diseases if the potential risk to the physician is small. If the risk is very substantial, physicians are not obligated to endanger their own lives. Historically, those who cared for patients during plagues were highly paid for their perilous work.

The commandment to visit the sick applies to everyone in cases in which there is little or no danger of contracting the illness from the patient. The risk to the average person of contracting hepatitis or AIDS by visiting a patient with these disorders is very small indeed. Hence, these patients should be visited and comforted.

May the one and only true Healer of the sick effect a complete recovery of all people suffering from a variety of diseases and illnesses through the hands of His messengers on earth, the human physicians. May the Lord cure all sickness from the face of the earth and may He send us the Messiah and rebuild the Holy Temple in Jerusalem, speedily in our days, Amen.

5

PRIORITIES IN MEDICINE: WHOM TO TREAT FIRST

Abraham S. Abraham, M.D.

The dilemma of whom to treat when there are insufficient resources for the treatment of all who are in need is not a new one. This dilemma also arises when treatment *can* be give to all, but decisions must be made on the basis of priority—even when the decision is not purely a medical one.

The Talmud (*Baba Metzia* 62a) sets forth a situation in which two people are on a journey and only one possesses a flask of water. If the circumstances are such that if both were to share the contents of the flask neither would survive—whereas if the water were consumed by one of the two, that person might reach safety—what are the travelers to do? Ben Petura opines that both should share the water, even if this meant that, as a consequence, both would die, because this would be preferable to one living at the expense of the other. Rabbi Akiva, on the other hand, on the basis of the verse "That thy brother may live with thee" (Leviticus 25:36), concludes that "your own life comes before that of another"; therefore the one who owns the flask of water may consume all of it in order to survive. In his commentary on this talmudic passage, Rabbi Isaiah Karelitz, known as Chazon Ish, says that if the flask belonged to a third person who did not need to drink, and there was only sufficient water for one of two others who would otherwise die of thirst, the owner may give the water to whichever one of the two he chooses.[1] This ruling is restricted to a situation in which the other two are of the same status (see the next paragraph); otherwise the water should be given in the order of priority specified in the ruling of the Mishnah (*Horayot* 3:7).

PRIORITIES IN JUDAISM

From this we learn that in a life-threatening situation, the order of priority—that is, which of two persons to save—is as follows: male before female (since men must observe a larger number of commandments[2]); a Priest (*cohen*) before a Levite; a Levite before an Israelite; a sage or scholar (*talmid chacham*) before an ignoramus (*am haaretz*), and so on. In a medical situation, this order of priority holds only if the two persons present themselves to the physician at the same time; preference should then be assigned in accordance with the Mishnah.[3] However, if the patients involved are of the same status, the physician may choose whom first to treat. (See also the writings of Rabbi Yaakov Emden.[4])

Furthermore, this order of priority holds true only if both patients have equal status in terms of their potential for survival. However, if one patient would certainly die if left untreated and the other only questionably, then the physician should first treat the patient who would otherwise certainly

---

1. Commentary on *Baba Metzia* 62a.
2. M. Maimonides, Commentary on the Mishnah, *Horayot* 3:7.
3. J. Karo, *Shulchan Aruch, Yoreh De'ah* 251:9.
4. *Migdal Oz, Even Bocher*, 1: 91–92.

die. Similarly, if one person has no chance (or only a very small chance) of surviving if treated, and the other has a good chance of surviving if treated, the latter should be given priority.[5]

Two questions must be asked. First, we know that the order of priority applies when both patients present at the same time to the physician who is in a position to treat only one of them. However, what would be the ruling if the two patients had arrived in the emergency room one *after* the other, but the physician had arrived later and found them both together? Does the rule of priority as stated in the Mishnah still hold, or should the physician first treat the patient who had arrived at the hospital first? In other words, should he proceed on the basis of "first come, first served"?

The problem of prioritization applies not *only* to patients in mortal danger, but also to situations in which two patients who are not seriously ill present simultaneously to the physician. Therefore, the foregoing question might be rephrased as follows: If a physician walks into his office and is confronted with a full waiting room, is it "first come, first served" (either on the basis of who arrived first or who had the first appointment), or is it the Priest before the Israelite, even though the Israelite has been waiting an hour and the Priest only five minutes? The same halachah (Jewish legal ruling) applies not only to the physician vis-à-vis patients, but also to the giving of charity or other acts of kindness,[6] or to the bank teller and the bank's clients or the shop attendant and the customers.[7]

Now the second question: Does anyone in practice

---

5. Y. Te'umim, *Pri Megadim*, commentary on *Orach Chayim* 328, section *Mishbetzot Zehav* 1; E. Y. Waldenberg, Responsa *Tzitz Eliezer*, vol. 9, no. 17:10:5 and no. 28:3; M. Feinstein, Responsa *Iggrot Moshe*, *Choshen Mishpat*, part 2, no. 73:2.

6. A. S. Abraham, *Nishmat Avraham*, *Yoreh De'ah* 252:2, cited in the name of Rabbi Shlomo Zalman Auerbach.

7. I. Lipschutz, commentary *Tiferet Yisrael* on *Horayot* 3:7, note 33.

observe the order of priority stated in the Mishnah? Does the physician do so with his patients? Does the rabbi so behave if he comes home to find people waiting to tell him their problems? The answer, obviously, is no! But why not? What justifies behavior contrary to the ruling of the Mishnah and the Code of Jewish law (*Shulchan Aruch*)?

This second question is asked by Rabbi Abraham Gumbiner,[8] in relation to the Priest's right to priority: Why is it that we do not find that he is given priority in the foregoing circumstances? Gumbiner's answer is that it is probably because of the questionability of the present-day Priest's being an indubitable and direct descendant of Aaron the High Priest.[9] This answer is also given by Rabbi Yaakov Emden.[10]

A parallel may be noted in the prioritization of men versus women. One possibility for consideration is based on the line of reasoning set forth by the Magen Avraham: The man has priority over the woman because he is commanded to observe, and we assume that he indeed *performs*, more commandments (*mitzvot*) than a woman. However, do we truly know which of the two patients *actually observes* more commandments? The Talmud (*Taanit* 23a) relates that when Abba Chilkiah and his wife prayed for rain, his wife's prayers were answered because she, being at home, had given already prepared food to the beggar at the door. Abba Chilkiah, on the other hand, had given money, with which the beggar then had to *buy* food. Similarly, the Talmud (*Ketubot* 67 b) relates how Mar Ukva was saved from danger by the greater merits of his wife.

With regard to a sage vis-à-vis an ignoramus, we are told (*Baba Bathra* 10b) that in the world to come, the teacher

---

8. Commentary *Magen Avraham* on J. Karo's *Shulchan Aruch, Orach Chayim* 201:4.

9. *Nishmat Avraham, Orach Chayim* 128:10, at the end.

10. Op. cit., part 1:89.

may find himself in a status lower than that of a former pupil.[11] In addition, some rabbinic authorities hold that nowadays no one complies with the definition of "sage" (*talmid chacham*) as required by the Talmud,[12] and that it could therefore be argued that today only a person who is outstanding in learning or piety should be given priority.

FIRST COME – FIRST SERVED PRINCIPLE

With regard to our first question, the *Shulchan Aruch* (*Choshen Mishpat* 15:1) states that if two cases are awaiting judgment, the *beth din* (court of law) should consider them in the order of their presentation, unless one involved a "sage." This ruling implies that even if the two cases were already waiting when the beth din convened, the rules of priority would apply. However, Rabbi Yosha' Valk Cohen,[13] known as the Sema, limits this ruling to a situation in which the parties appear *after* the *beth din* had already convened; only then does the "first come–first served" rule apply. However, those already waiting *before* the convening of the *beth din* are subject to the standard rules of prioritization even if one arrived before the other, and the *beth din* may choose to deal first with whichever case it wishes (unless one involves a sage).

Rabbi Waldenberg[14] has stated that this ruling of *Shulchan Aruch* is not generally accepted and that many authorities, foremost among them Rashi, Maimonides (Rambam), and Tosafot, decided that, on the contrary, the sage's priority

---

11. Commentary of Tosafot on *Baba Bathra* 10b, s. v. *elyonim*.

12. M. Isserles, glossary known as *Ramah* on J. Karo's *Shulchan Aruch*, *Yoreh De'ah* 243:2 and 243:7; A. Z. Eisenstadt, commentary *Pitchei Teshuvah*, ibid., 243:2:2; M. L. Avraham, commentary *Yad Avraham*, ibid.; *Mishnah Berurah* 547:12.

13. Ibid. 15:1:1.

14. Personal communication.

applies only if he arrived together with the ignoramus. Therefore, the answer to the foregoing question depends upon a combination of two propositions: (1) Whether the Mishnah applies only to the situation in which the two patients (the sage and the ignoramus) presented simultaneously to the physician, or whether the Mishnah is relevant if the parties arrived at different times and the physician arrived to find them both waiting; and (2) whether anyone in modern times can rightly be called a sage. A combination of these two doubts (*safek sefekah*) explains why the priorities set forth in the Mishnah are no longer adhered to today. Rabbi Waldenberg, however, is of the opinion that a recognized "sage" or person of outstanding piety should be given priority even if that person arrives after the physician has already started consultation hours.

The question of what significance "waiting in line" has in Halachah in terms of giving preference to the first in line (even when those in line are all of equal status) is also not clear. Rabbi Waldenberg writes that this is only a custom hallowed by public consent, and that it therefore cannot override Halachah as enunciated in the Mishnah. Rabbi Yitzchak Zilberstein[15] quotes Rabbi Menachem Meiri,[16] who suggests that "first come, first served" is not merely custom, but is supported by the verse "Justice, justice shalt thou pursue" (Deuteronomy 16:20); therefore, such priority should prevail as long as it does not contradict the Halachah of the Mishnah.

Finally, Rabbi Moshe Feinstein[17] writes that although priorities should be assigned only according to the criteria cited in the Mishnah, it would be difficult to apply them in practice without great deliberation.

15. *Halachah Urefuah*, vol. 3, ed. M. Hershler (Jerusalem, 1983), pp. 91–101.
16. Commentary *Meiri* (*Bet Habechirah*) on *Sanhedrin* 32b.
17. *Responsa Iggrot Moshe, Choshen Mishpat*, part 2, 74:1.

CONCLUSIONS

All the conclusions reached thus far apply only to the situation in which the physician has not actually started to treat the patient. If treatment is already underway, such treatment may not be interrupted in favor of another patient. This rule applies to treatment by the physician personally as well as to the use of equipment for treatment, such as an intensive care unit bed or a respirator. In such a situation, regardless of the medical or other status of the two patients, nothing is permitted that may result in the sacrifice of the patient who is already being treated, in favor of the other. Thus, if interrupting treatment would mean the earlier death of an elderly, chronically ill patient who would be expected to die even in spite of continuing treatment, interruption of treatment is still forbidden, even in order to save the viable life of another person who is young and intrinsically healthy. As Rabbi Shlomo Zalman Auerbach says:[18] One may not sacrifice a life for a life, even to save oneself, or even to save the life of a person of outstanding learning and piety and who serves the world at large, by means which hasten the death of a person who may be very aged, mentally incapacitated, and a burden to others.

---

18. Cited in *Nishmat Avraham, Yoreh De'ah* 252:2.

6

THE PATIENT ON THE SABBATH

Abraham S. Abraham, M.D.

Halachah recognizes four categories of illness to correspond to the practical implications regarding the Sabbath, Yom Kippur, Passover, forbidden foods, and so on. In this chapter I will discuss in general terms when, under what circumstances, and by whom the Torah or rabbinic prohibitions may be set aside on the Sabbath on behalf of a patient. If at all possible, nothing should be done for a sick person on the Sabbath without prior consultation with a recognized rabbinic authority, to whom all the medical data should be presented in detail. There is one case of exception, in which it would indeed be wrong to seek such prior advice, and this is the case of a dangerously ill person who needs *immediate* medical attention and whose potential for recovery might be diminished by any delay in obtaining the required assistance (as described later in this chapter).

FOUR CATEGORIES OF ILLNESS

1. **Discomfort** *(meychush be'alma)*. Examples of this category include mild colds, mild coughs, or skin eruptions not

97

severe enough to affect the whole body.[1] A person with such symptoms should neither take medication nor receive treatment on the Sabbath,[2] even if this involves a prohibition of rabbinic origin alone,[3] and even if the treatment is administered by a non-Jew.[4] However, if the treatment is of such a nature that it would normally be administered even to healthy persons—for example, the use of a hot-water bottle—then the sick person may avail himself of it, even if this is not his custom when in a healthy state.[5]

2. Minor illness *(choleh bemiktzat* or *mitztayer harbeh).*[6] Examples of this category include a nasal catarrh, an irritating cough, or a headache that is severe but not severe enough to require bed rest. A person suffering from such an ailment may not *receive* treatment from a Jew that involves desecration of the Sabbath, even if it is a prohibition by rabbinic ordinance; nor may the patient *take* medicaments. The patient may be treated by a non-Jew, however, if such treatment involves a prohibition of rabbinic origin only.[7] Thus, it is permitted, for instance, to ask a non-Jew to bring food or medication, such as nose drops or eye drops, to be instilled by a non-Jew, even if they must be carried through areas that are not classified as public domain *(karmelit).* (See also Rabbi Josef Karo's *Shulchan Aruch.*[8])

3A. The severely but not fatally ill patient *(choleh she'ayn bo sakanah).* This category includes a number of subcategories:

---

1. I. M. Kagan, *Mishnah Berurah* 328:1.

2. J. Karo, *Shulchan Aruch, Orach Chayim* 328:1.

3. *Mishnah Berurah* 328:2.

4. Ibid., 328:3 and 328:100.

5. Y. Y. Neuwirth, *Shemirat Shabbat Kehilchatah,* chapter 34:11.

6. I. Lipschutz, Commentary *Tiferet Yisrael* in *Kilkelet Shabbat, Dinei Amirah Lenochri,* vol. 7, no. 1.

7. *Shulchan Aruch, Orach Chayim* 307:5; *Mishnah Berurah* 328:52.

8. M. Isserles, Glossary known as *Ramah* on the *Shulchan Aruch, Orach Chayim* 328:17.

(a) A person who is confined to bed or whose entire body is affected by illness or pain,[9] even if he is not seriously ill. Examples would be the patient with influenza or severe migraine.

(b) A person who, even if not confined to bed, is in a condition in which most others if similarly afflicted would take to bed.[10]

(c) A person who is prone to such an illness (for example, severe migraine) unless given preventive treatment.[11]

(d) A child of up to 2 or 3 years of age (depending on the stage of development),[12] even if suffering from only a mild illness.[13]

(e) A woman who is 8 to 30 days postpartum.[14]

For these categories of patients, a non-Jew may be instructed to carry out whatever treatment is necessary, even if this involves setting aside Torah prohibitions applicable to Jews.[15] In addition, a Jew may perform whatever tasks are necessary for the patient's care, provided that this is a prohibition of rabbinic ordinance and that the care is provided in a manner that differs from the ordinary procedure.[16] There is no need to seek a non-Jew to provide this care.[17] If a right-handed person uses his left hand to write on the Sabbath, this is considered as differing from ordinary procedure (*shinuy*), thus converting a biblical prohibition into a less stringent rabbinic one.[18]

---

9. Ibid.

10. Ibid.

11. S. Z. Auerbach, personal communication.

12. *Shemirat Shabbat Kehilchatah*, chapter 37:2.

13. *Ramah*, op. cit., 328:17.

14. *Shulchan Aruch, Orach Chayim* 330:4; *Shemirat Shabbat Kehilchatah*, chapter 36:15.

15. *Mishnah Berurah* 328:47.

16. Ibid., 328:57.

17. Ibid., 328:54.

18. A. Danzig, *Chayei Adam*, principle 9:2, cited in *Mishnah Berurah* 340:122, at the end.

If the patient or attendant cannot perform the tasks necessary for treatment other than by the ordinary methods, then the treatment may be performed in the normal manner, provided that the act is prohibited only by rabbinic ordinance.[19] This rule applies not only to the taking of medication, but also to any procedure that is necessary for the patient's welfare and that is of rabbinic prohibition only.[20]

In the context of the kinds of patients we have been discussing—those who are ill but not fatally so—some additional situations merit discussion:

(a) *The performance of an act prohibited by the Torah in a manner differing from the ordinary.* Rabbi Israel Meir Kagan[21] forbids such an act, but other authorities permit it.[22] Rabbi Shlomo Zalman Auerbach ruled that since these recognized authorities hold that this act is permitted, their opinion should prevail if a non-Jew is not available to perform the procedure that is prohibited by the Torah. Consider, for example, the ill person who visits a Jewish physician on the Sabbath and realizes that the physician is about to perform an act ordinarily prohibited by the Torah but necessary for diagnosis or treatment (such as switching on the light). If the patient is unable to persuade the physician to perform the necessary act in a manner other than that which is usual, then the patient himself should, if possible, apply the unusual procedure, in preference to the physician's performing the act in the usual fashion.[23]

(b) *An act that is performed for a purpose other than that for*

---

19. *Mishnah Berurah* 328:102, cited in the name of the *Chayei Adam*.

20. *Shemirat Shabbat Kehilchatah*, chapter 33, note 23.

21. *Mishnah Berurah* 496, in note *Sha'ar HaSion* 9.

22. Shneur Zalman of Ladi, *Shulchan Aruch Harav* 328:19; David Ortenberg, *Tehilah leDavid* 328:22; Avraham Sokachov, *Igle Tal*, chapter *Melechet Tochen* 17:38(10); Avraham Chaim Noeh, *Ketsot Hashulchan* 134:4 in note *Bade Hashulchan* 6.

23. *Shemirat Shabbat Kehilchatah*, chapter 33, note 17.

which it was used in the Tabernacle (melachah she'aynah tzerichah legufah). An example of such an act is the extinguishing of burning material, which was performed in the Tabernacle (*Mishkan*) only for the purpose of making charcoal. Thus, extinguishing light in order to allow a patient to sleep is, according to many authorities, a prohibition that is by rabbinic ordinance. According to Maimonides, however, it is a prohibition of the Torah and therefore may not be set aside for a generally, but not fatally, ill person.[24]

3B. Danger to a limb but not to life. Karo's ruling in the *Shulchan Aruch* is that in the event of danger to a limb but not to life, a non-Jew may be asked to do whatever is necessary for the patient's welfare, even if such an act is prohibited by the Torah.[25] In such cases a Jew is allowed to perform only those acts that are prohibited only by rabbinic ordinance, but these acts may be performed by standard methods.[26] Nevertheless, if there is no danger to life as a consequence of withholding treatment, a Jew may not transgress a prohibition of the Torah.[27] An exception to this rule is the case in which there is danger of loss of an eye or sight; in such a case a Jew may do whatever is necessary for the patient, even if such an act would otherwise be prohibited by the Torah.[28]

When there is danger to a limb, the law is more lenient than it is for a patient in category 3A. Thus, the following rules apply: First, one may carry out an act otherwise forbidden by the Torah as long as one does so by a procedure *other than* the ordinary one; there is no need in such a case to

---

24. *Mishnah Berurah* 278:3; see also *Shemirat Shabbat Kehilchatah*, chapter 33, note 22.

25. *Shulchan Aruch, Orach Chayim* 328:17, in the third opinion.

26. *Mishnah Berurah* 328:57.

27. Ibid., 328:49.

28. *Shulchan Aruch, Orach Chayim* 328:9; *Mishnah Berurah* 328:22.

seek the assistance of a non-Jew.[29] And second, an act performed for a purpose other than its original intent in the Tabernacle—see item (b) on pages 100–101—is permitted.[30]

Rabbi Avraham Chaim Noeh[31] interprets the ruling of the *Shulchan Aruch* to cover not only the physical loss of a limb or its loss of function but also its loss of *normal* function (for example, in paresis, as opposed to paralysis, of a hand or leg).[32] According to Rabbi Yehoshua Neuwirth, one may further extend this decision to apply not only to a limb but also to any organ of the body that, if left untreated, would not function satisfactorily. Thus, if the function of the uterus and ovaries for conception and pregnancy might be affected without appropriate treatment, such a state is included in the ruling concerning danger to a limb.[33]

4. The patient suffering from a potentially fatal condition (*choleh sheyesh bo sakanah*). According to the talmudic commentary known as Tosafot (*Yoma* 85a), no treatment may be withheld if withholding it could conceivably lead to the death of a patient. This category includes the following:

(a) A patient who senses the serious nature of his illness,[34] or a patient whose physician[35] (or any other person with some knowledge of medicine)[36] states that the illness is serious. If there is a difference of opinion between the physician and the patient, the more stringent opinion pre-

---

29. *Shemirat Shabbat Kehilchatah*, chapter 33, note 17, cited in the name of Rabbi Shlomo Zalman Auerbach.
30. Ibid.
31. *Ketsot Hashulchan* 138, in note *Bade Hashulchan* 18, at the end.
32. Also cited in *Shemirat Shabbat Kehilchatah*, chapter 33:1, note 5.
33. Y. Y. Neuwirth, personal communication.
34. *Shulchan Aruch, Orach Chayim* 328:5.
35. Ibid., 328:10.
36. *Mishnah Berurah* 328:27 and 328:28.

vails even if it is that of the patient and even if it is contrary to the judgment of the physician.[37]

(b) A patient who, although not in immediate danger, may deteriorate into such a state unless given treatment in time.[38] An example of such a patient is the brittle insulin-dependent diabetic who has run out of insulin.

(c) Patients with certain conditions ruled by the Talmud to be states of danger, even if they are not considered dangerous according to current medical opinion.[39] An example is a woman who is up to 7 days postpartum.[40]

There are two basic situations that could pertain to patients in the fourth category (i.e., those whose illness is potentially fatal). The first is the situation in which there is imminent or *potentially* imminent danger to life.[41] In such a case, one must do everything necessary to save life as quickly as possible, exactly as one would do if it were not the Sabbath.[42] One who delays treatment in such a situation in order first to seek a rabbinic decision is considered to have "shed blood," since the delay may result in loss of life.[43]

The second situation is that in which it is *certain* that there will be no imminent danger to life if one does not act immediately. In such a situation, time should be taken to consult a competent rabbinic authority in order to obtain guidance on when and how to set aside the Sabbath.

---

37. *Mishnah Berurah (Be'ur Halachah)* 328:10, s.v. *Verofeh*; *Shemirat Shabbat Kehilchatah*, chapter 32:9.

38. *Mishnah Berurah* 328:17; *Shulchan Aruch, Orach Chayim* 321:18 and *Mishnah Berurah* 321:75; *Shemirat Shabbat Kehilchatah*, chapter 32:8.

39. *Mishnah Berurah* 328:8.

40. *Shulchan Aruch, Orach Chayim* 330:4.

41. *Mishnah Berurah* 328:17.

42. *Shulchan Aruch, Orach Chayim* 328:2 and 328:5.

43. Ibid., 328:2 and 328:13; *Mishnah Berurah* 328:6.

CONCLUSIONS

For physicians, nurses, and medical attendants who have to
face these problems every Sabbath, there is no substitute for
studying the rules of Sabbath in general, and the rules
concerning patients in particular, with a competent teacher.
The duties of caring for patients can then be carried out most
correctly and efficiently in accordance with halachic principles.

7

CONTRACEPTION AND ABORTION

Rabbi Moshe D. Tendler, Ph.D.

The halachic–medical interface at the beginning of life impinges upon the daily practice of medicine. Therefore, much of this chapter is strictly in the realm of practical Halachah. I offer the following caution: A book chapter should not substitute for the classic technique of *sho'el umeshiv*, whereby one asks a halachic question and receives an answer from a competent rav. In this way, Halachah is clarified for one's personal and professional life. The key references include the Talmud (*Yebamot* 75), the Code of Jewish Law,[1] and the various responsa that are referred to in this chapter, including those of Rabbi Isaiah Karelitz[2] and Rabbi Moshe Feinstein.[3]

---

1. J. Karo, *Shulchan Aruch, Even Haezer* 5:1ff.
2. *Responsa Chazon Ish, Even Haezer*, no. 12:13.
3. *Responsa Iggrot Moshe, Even Haezer*, part 3, nos. 12, 13; part 4, no. 30.

VASECTOMY AS A METHOD OF CONTRACEPTION

The prohibition of sterilization as a method of contraception needs attention. It is to me the prime proof of the spotty nature of Torah education. How is it possible for an observant Jew who observes the Sabbath and the laws of family purity and who eats *glat* kosher to undergo a vasectomy because his physician believed it to be the wisest method of contraception for his family? It obviously never occurred to this Jew that this is an area for halachic concern. One of the curriculum problems in Torah education in our day school and Yeshiva system is that we fail to adequately inculcate our students with the truism that no area of human concern is devoid of halachic guidelines. In every class it is taught that one must not touch a candlestick on the Sabbath because it is prohibited as *muktzah*. Yet young students are never taught that one must not injure oneself or touch someone else's wallet, or spouse. Vasectomy leads to *pesul kahal*; in other words, a man who has undergone a vasectomy must divorce his wife and may then never marry a woman born in the Jewish faith. There is no permissibility (*heter*) for vasectomy in Judaism other than to save the life of a patient. Consequently, the use of vasectomy is an unthinkable method of contraception for the Jewish community.

In addition, the prohibition against sterilization is a negative precept in the Torah (*Lo Taaseh*). A religious Jew should not become a veterinarian. The bread–and–butter business of the veterinarian (especially in an urban area) is the castration or spaying of small animals. Therefore, a Torah-observant Jew cannot earn a living by being a veterinarian in such a setting.

There is a well-known responsum from my late father-in-law Rabbi Moshe Feinstein, of blessed memory, which, based upon *Chazon Ish*, states that the surgical interruption of the *vas deferens* that occurs during prostatectomy does not present a significant halachic problem. (In fact, with the use of current surgical technique, such interruption is often not involved at all.) Nevertheless, it is interesting to note the development of that responsum of the Chazon Ish[4] in which he describes the anatomy of the male reproductive tract and sets the limits of the prohibition of sterilization or castration (*seerus*).

Of more practical concern for our times is the issue of what is to be done after someone has already *had* a vasectomy. Here we have a spinoff of the *Ba'al Teshuvah*[5] movement of which many are not aware. I have addressed over ninety questions related to this issue—questions asked by Jewish physicians and their Jewish patients who have undergone vasectomy. We lived during the 1960s through a strange period of the "flower children," who knew not the Torah received at Mount Sinai but only the moral chaos inherited from their parents (Jeremiah 16:19). These young men and women joined communes and set up their own regulations, their own "Torah." It was quite common for these men to be vasectomized, for they believed that this world was no place to bring more children into being.

God helped many of these people to return to the religion of their ancestors, and late in their repentant experience they discovered the terrible consequence of what they had perpetrated. Applicable in this context is an important responsum from Rabbi Feinstein,[6] in which he pointed out the novel rabbinic concept that intent and purpose can modify the rabbinic interpretation of a prohibited act. There is a prohibition against castration after castration or sterilization after sterilization (*seerus* after *seerus*). A reverse vasectomy can be performed only by cutting into the *vas deferens* again to reach live tissue in order to make the anastamosis.

---

4. *Responsa Chazon Ish*, loc. cit.
5. Literally, a repentant person; i.e., one who became an Orthodox Jew.
6. *Responsa Iggrot Moshe*, part 4, no. 30.

The second act of cutting is prohibited, just as the initial act of the vasectomy was. Indeed, if a patient had undergone a vasectomy, was concerned that it had not been performed properly, and visited a second doctor to have the procedure redone, the second doctor would be transgressing the prohibition against sterilization just as the first one had. Similarly, in the repair (or *reversal*) process, the physician has no choice but to add to the initial vasectomy surgery by removing another section of the *vas deferens* and then employing a microsurgical technique to attempt to reanastamose the two ends. However, Rabbi Feinstein reached the conclusion that reanastamosis of the severed ends of the *vas deferens* would reestablish the eligibility of these Jewish men to marry within the Jewish faith. It is probable that most of my referrals for reanastamosis (sometimes called revasectomy) come from the *Ba'al Teshuvah* movement.

Rabbi Feinstein has further observed that after the *vas deferens* is revasectomized—in *reverse* vasectomy—the duct may be patent but, for reasons not fully understood, it is often difficult for the patient to impregnate his wife. This problem may be associated with antibodies that accumulated during the time that the sperm were not finding easy access or due to mechanical damage at the point of reanastamosis. The reality, however, is that the state of infertility often persists. Based upon his earlier responsum on prostatectomy,[7] Rabbi Feinstein stated that since the anatomical alteration was corrected, we cannot assume that inability to conceive is evidence that the reanastamosis was unsuccessful. Rather, the infertility is considered similar to that which occurs in men who have never undergone vasectomy. Therefore, the problem should be treated just as any case of infertility would be, without any subsequent prohibition of marrying within the Jewish faith.

---

7. Ibid., nos. 28–29.

TUBAL LIGATION AS A METHOD OF CONTRACEPTION

Tubal ligation has become a widely used method of surgical contraception within the Orthodox Jewish community. The Jewish laity and, regrettably, even some community rabbis are not familiar with the pertinent halachah. The prohibition of sterilization evoked a difference of opinion between Rabbi Elijah of Vilna, known as the Vilna Gaon, and the early talmudic commentators known as *rishonim*. The Vilna Gaon, in his commentary on the *Shulchan Aruch*,[8] specifically declares that the sterilization of a woman is a violation of a positive commandment in the Bible (*Issure Aseh*). The rishonim, on the other hand, refer to it as only a rabbinic prohibition. This difference of opinion is of great consequence in terms of the practical application of Halachah to actual cases. In the case of a specific family problem that is a source of great anguish and that cannot be resolved by other contraceptive means, one might consider tubal ligation as an option if sterilization is only a rabbinic prohibition. If it is a biblical prohibition, however, the rabbis would not be prepared to permit it.

This is the basis of the difference of opinion among the rabbinic decisors as to whether or not tubal ligation should be permitted under specific circumstances. Halachah sanctions tubal ligation in actual practice only when there is significant stress on the woman, leading to serious psychological disturbances that affect the family's life, or when there is significant medical reason, such as kidney failure or severe cardiac insufficiency such that pregnancy might be life-threatening. If it can be determined with absolute certainty that the patient must not become pregnant, then tubal ligation may be considered, but it is not a method of first choice under any condition.

---

8. *Shulchan Aruch, Even Haezer* 5:25.

All too often it happens that a couple decides not to have any more children, and, because of the vicissitudes of fate, a new family is suddenly involved. Perhaps the husband dies or the couple divorces, and the woman subsequently remarries. The birth of a child would add significantly to the bonding of the newly married couple, but if the woman has undergone a tubal ligation she probably will not be able to conceive. Hence, it is proper to discourage as much as possible any definitive procedure such as surgical interruption of the fallopian tubes. Although it is sometimes possible to reanastamose the severed tubes, the potential for success is extremely limited.

Of special interest are some of the newer techniques that are being tested on an experimental basis. One such procedure is "intentional reverse vasectomy," for which a temporary or reversible technique is used. Our example is the silicone plug, which involves the use of a valve that can be turned on and off, or that works on a magnetic switch that can be activated or deactivated by an external magnetic force. Such procedures involve intriguing halachic problems pertaining to the basic definition of the prohibition of *seerus*. Sterilization or castration that does not lead to infertility is not defined as *seerus*. *Seerus* that reverses itself—that is, in which "the closure opens"[9]—also carries no halachic consequences. What is the position of Jewish law if a physician intentionally performs a surgical procedure that is temporary—that can be reversed or turned on and off at will? Is that procedure subsumed under the prohibition of *seerus*? I know of no definitive responsum on this question.

Another new technique was reported by a team of investigators who showed for the first time the ease with which an individual with a congential absence of the *vas deferens* can indeed father a child.[10] They reported a series of

---

9. Ibid., 5:4.
10. P. Patrizio, S. Silbek, T. Ord, et al., "Two Births after Microsurgical

eight cases, in seven of which they successfully removed sperm from the testis itself using a technique known as zonal drilling. The investigators inserted the sperm into the ova of the patients' wives, and produced viable offspring from these in vitro fertilizations. These successful cases seem to violate biological rules concerning sperm capacitation, sperm maturation during passage through the *vas deferens*, and so on. Nevertheless, the babies were born.

This study evokes an interesting rabbinic question with practical application because one must perform an act of "halachic castration" during the procedure. These physicians actually cut into the rudimentary existing *vas deferens*, which is an act of *seerus*; but the purpose of the act is to overcome infertility. Hence, one must again apply Rabbi Feinstein's principle that if the goal of the act is the opposite of intentional castration, one cannot assign to it the halachic consequences that follow from an act of *seerus*.

This topic will require practical halachic decisions. Since the report was published I have referred several people for this procedure. For some unknown reason, the incidence of congenital absence of the *vas deferens* is disproportionately high in the Orthodox Jewish community, almost as if there were some factor in our lifestyle that predisposes us to that condition.

HORMONAL CONTRACEPTION

Hormonal contraception is the method most widely used by Jews and non-Jews alike. How does one approach this topic? This subject is widely discussed in the Orthodox or yeshiva community among young newlyweds. Such couples have innovated a modern definition of *frumkeit* (piety). They are

Sperm Aspiration in Congenital Absence of *Vas Deferens*," *Lancet*, vol. 2 (1988), p. 1364.

committed to the halachic process but want to know "the least minimal prohibition." Planning to use contraceptives anyway, they ask the rabbi, "Please tell me what is the smallest prohibition in regard to contraception?" This is an American–type question that I am sure no European rabbi was ever asked. In the United States there is a special charm to being "frank" and "open." In Europe it was called *chutzpah* (temerity).

The use of exogenous hormones to interrupt the menstrual cycle as a means of inducing a nonovulatory state is approached halachically with a simple checklist. First, as in the case of any new procedure, a risk–benefit analysis must be applied. Is the use of oral contraception allowed because there is a possible danger to health? Here we have a difference of opinion among members of the medical profession. Several reviews of the association between cervical[11] and breast cancer[12] and the use of oral contraceptives have concluded that there is a threefold increase in these cancers among women who take the pill (both invasive cancer and carcinoma-in-situ). Other studies also support the fact that there is an increase in the incidence of breast cancer following the use of oral contraceptives. The halachic prohibitions against intentionally injuring oneself or endangering one's health or life must be considered.

The halachic question concerns risk–benefit ratios as well as motivation. What is the reason for the use of oral contraceptives? If the reason is adequate, then the risk might be an acceptable one under the broad principle of *doshu bo rabim*, or societal acceptance. Since so many people accept this modicum of risk, it should be looked upon not as

11. V. Beral, P. Hannaford, C. Kay, "Oral Contraceptive Use and Malignancies of the Genital Tract: Results from the Royal College of General Practitioners' Oral Contraception Study," *Lancet*, vol. 2 (1988), pp. 1331–1335.

12. UK National Case-Control Study Group, "Oral Contraceptive Use and Breast Cancer Risk in Young Women," *Lancet*, vol. 1 (1989), pp. 973–982.

self-harm but only as one of the many risks faced by mortal humans in the course of daily life.

Research has produced conflicting results on the question of whether the oral contraceptive pill reduces the incidence of ovarian cancer and cervical cancer. The latter issue is not too relevant to the Orthodox Jewish community because cervical cancer apparently does not affect Orthodox women. It is of great historical and theological significance that we have yet to record a single proven case of a woman who observed the laws of family purity and yet developed cervical cancer. Ovarian cancer, on the other hand, afflicts both Jewish and non-Jewish women. An increased incidence of blood-clotting disorders, including pulmonary emboli, in women taking the contraceptive pill is also noteworthy in evaluating the risk associated with these drugs.

Hence, in assessing whether or not it is permissible to use oral contraception, one must take into account more than just the question of contraception, which itself is a thwarting of the positive commandment of procreation. In Judaism, when a young couple marries, they are supposed to have children. The commandment to be fruitful should not be delayed, as is the rule with any *mitzvah* (commandment) incumbent on a Jew. This is one of the controversial areas of Halachah in which the rabbi must evaluate each case individually. Here, the method of contraception becomes critical because, as the halachic objections to a contraceptive method increase, the significance of the reasons for using the method must increase as well. Therefore, in most circumstances, the contraceptive method to be recommended, if there is a halachic reason to consider contraception, is the oral contraceptive as this is associated with "the least minimal prohibition." The health factors previously mentioned must be factored into this equation.

The idea of justifying the temporary use of contraception so that the couple can "get to know each other" before they have children has become widely accepted within the

Orthodox community. I would suggest instead that the couple wait a few years before they marry. It is not advisable to marry somebody one does not know. There is no permissibility to use contraception without valid cause. There is no permissibility for a bride who wants to regulate her menstrual cycle to be on birth control pills during the month in which she gets married. If she wants to regulate her cycle, she must do so during the previous month. During the month of her marriage, she must be on her natural cycle, not on an artificial cycle induced by an oral contraceptive. To do otherwise requires a permissive rabbinic ruling, and such a ruling should not be granted under normal circumstances.

Another issue that causes much confusion is the problem of intermenstrual "spotting" caused by the oral contraceptive pill. The manufacturers of these drugs cite a low incidence of intermenstrual bleeding. Regrettably, some rabbis have assumed that this bleeding is unrelated to the halachic concept of *nidah*, whereby a woman is not permitted to cohabit with her husband if she bleeds even one drop of blood. But such bleeding, although intermenstrual, does in fact put her in the status of *nidah*. If a woman taking the pill were to visit her physician and say, "I looked and I found a pin-prick-sized blood spot," the physician would say, "Do not bother me. That drop of blood is not a medical issue." Such minor bleeding is not recorded in the investigational data on the pill and is not reported to the drug manufacturer because it is deemed medically insignificant. In Halachah, however, no distinction is made between active bleeding and the spilling of one drop of blood; in both cases, the woman is classified in the status of *nidah* and must undergo ritual purification in a ritualarium (*mikveh*) after the prescribed time period before she can again cohabit with her husband. The incidence of such spotting in women taking oral contraceptives may be as high as 60 percent. If a woman on the pill makes the effort to examine herself at least once a day all month long, she will never be able to go to the *mikveh*.

She cannot say "I will not look," because she is doing something to induce the state of *nidah*. She must examine herself daily during the first three months in which she is taking the pill. By the fourth month, the spotting generally ceases. Therefore, a woman who is using oral contraception must examine herself twice daily for the first three months, after which she may establish the presumption (*chazakah*) that her endometrium now resembles that of a postmenopausal woman and that she will no longer be subject to bleeding.

Of special concern is a new issue of which I have become aware because many physicians refer their patients to me with halachic questions relating to *nidah*. Nursing women are now being given progesterone-containing contraceptive agents because estrogens interfere with the nursing. They take only progesterone. When they report to their physicians that they are staining, the physicians tell them that it is a result of the nursing and is of no consequence. However, this bleeding renders the woman a *nidah*. Therefore, as contraceptive agents that contain only progesterone almost invariably cause bleeding, they may not be used by Orthodox Jewish women.

Progesterone-containing contraceptive agents are prescribed by physicians for nursing women who do not want to become pregnant again or who have previously become pregnant even while nursing. An interesting halachic analysis of a medical study in which progesterones were administered parenterally every three to six months is found in the responsa of Rabbi Feinstein.[13] He refers to both the castration (*seerus*) aspect, since women could not become pregnant for six months, and the *nidah,* or ritual impurity aspect of this contraceptive modality.

---

13. *Responsa Iggrot Moshe, Even Haezer* 1:62–63, 3:12.

CHEMICAL CONTRACEPTION

In three separate responsa,[14] Rabbi Feinstein equates the use of spermicidal agents with the use of the pill. He analyzes the attitude of the Sages toward medically indicated contraception as follows: This method is not looked upon as a mechanical barrier but strictly as a means of establishing an environment that is inimical to the sperm, no different from the oral contraceptive "potion" described in the Talmud and no different from the contraceptive pill. Therefore, whenever the pill can be used, spermicidal agents may also be used.

MECHANICAL CONTRACEPTION

The use of the diaphragm, contraceptive sponge, and cervical cap is permitted only if the woman has a significant medical problem. In the absence of a medical problem—physiological or psychiatric—the use of any of the mechanical barriers is prohibited even though the mechanical barriers require the addition of a spermicidal agent to enhance their effectiveness. Rabbi Akiba Eger ruled that the use of the diaphragm is not permissible, even in the case of danger to the life of the patient if she were to become pregnant.[15]

Some of our rabbis have understood that there is an alternative to contraception. Why look for a permissive ruling? They suggested a simple solution: Do not have sexual relations. If there is a problem regarding contraception, why not just decide that it is prohibited? If one were to be in an area that had no *mikveh*, one would not seek a permissive ruling to allow cohabitation when one's wife is a *nidah*. It is prohibited, period! Thus, if pregnancy would be life-threatening, why not require abstinence? No contemporary rabbinic authority suggests such an approach, however,

---

14. Ibid.
15. *Responsa Rabbi Akiba Eger*, no. 71.

because the talmudic Sages mandated (or at least allowed) the use of a mechanical barrier in the case of three types of women for whom pregnancy might be dangerous (*Yebamot* 12b). It apparently never occurred to the Sages to suggest that it is possible that a married state should exist without the bond being reinforced by the marital act. Rabbi Feinstein deduces therefrom that we must find permissive rulings for these questions, but that these permissive rulings must be within the strict limits of Halachah and not derived from secular rationalizations. Therefore, contraceptive techniques are not all equally acceptable or unacceptable in Halachah. The use of a mechanical barrier as a method of contraception is permitted only for medical reasons.

The intrauterine device (IUD) merits special note. Because of the medical problems associated with a particular brand of IUD, only two forms of the device are currently available. The IUD should not be used by women who observe Halachah because the IUD causes spot bleeding throughout the menstrual cycle. Although this spotting is said to be due to an inflammatory response to the presence of the IUD in the uterine lining, Halachah states that any spotting must be treated as rendering the woman *nidah*.

ABORTION AND ITS TECHNOLOGIES

The prohibition against abortion is clear; it is one of the seven Noahide commandments. The Bible states: "Whosoever sheddeth the blood of man in man, his blood shall be shed" (Genesis 9:6). The phrase "man in man" is interpreted to refer to a fetus (*Sanhedrin* 57b). Rabbi Feinstein wrote very strongly on this point.[16] He ruled that abortion defies the prohibition of killing. Although this prohibition was com-

---

16. *Sefer Hazikaron LehaGaon R. Yechezkel Abramsky* (memorial volume to R. Yechezkel Abramsky, 1978 [5738]).

municated primarily to the sons of Noah (i.e., non-Jews), the prohibition against killing a fetus also applies to Jews.

It is not permissible according to Jewish law to destroy a fetus, except in the classic rabbinic situation of the *rodef* (literally, "pursuer"), who is threatening the life of another. Such a person must be stopped even if it means killing him, in order to thwart the danger to the person being pursued. A pregnant woman whose life is in danger, physiologically or psychologically, may have an abortion to eliminate the threat to her life. A suicidal woman who accidentally became pregnant has the same permissibility as someone whose pregnancy physically endangers her life. If the woman has end-stage renal disease or some similarly life-threatening disorder, abortion should be performed if continued pregnancy would endanger her life.

Of great moral concern is the "preparation to transgress." Amniocentesis, chorionic villus sampling, and embryo biopsy are all directed to abortion and no other purpose. Gene therapy and fetal surgery are too poorly developed to justify the use of these prenatal procedures at this time. One cannot justify the abortion of a child who might be born handicapped by considering it to be for the child's benefit, let alone for the benefit of the woman. The "perfect child" bias is built into our society. Most mothers who might be given the option of abortion by a physician who said, "Your unborn child has a cleft lip," will expend considerable effort to determine whether or not to abort. Such questions are often posed to a rabbi for a *psak* (rabbinic ruling). The "perfect child" bias insists that all our children be flawless. The fact that a child with a cleft lip could grow up to be a great talmudic scholar and a happy, contented adult is not always considered by those who cling to an idyllic image of what the mortal world holds for them. Therefore, if a woman undergoes one of the aforementioned procedures and discovers that something is wrong with her child, the drive to abort may be irresistible.

Amniocentesis and/or ultrasound examination are now routinely done in early pregnancy. Detection by the physician of even a slight aberration in the ultrasound image is sufficient to evoke severe anxiety in the patient. Many women in this situation fail the test of discipline and opt for abortion. Consequently, amniocentesis or ultrasound examination without specific medical indication should be strongly discouraged.

These procedures may now also be performed for the purpose of sex selection. If a couple have two sons and wish to know the sex of their unborn child, they can obtain the information by amniocentesis, or sometimes by ultrasound, and may react with a decision to abort. Consequently, amniocentesis should be looked upon as what it is: part of the abortion technology system.

The risk of inducing abortion by amniocentesis is also a factor in the halachic evaluation. About 1 percent of women spontaneously abort as a consequence of amniocentesis, even if the child would have been perfectly normal.

One use of ultrasound examination in an abortion clinic is of particular interest. Several hundred young women who presented for abortion early in pregnancy underwent ultrasound examination.[17] Some of these women were allowed to see the ultrasound images. They were able to see that there was "something there." Other women, who did not see the ultrasound images, went through with their planned abortions. However, many of those who watched the procedure and saw the humanoid form of the fetus did not go through with their abortions. Ultrasound may thus be used not only to provide information that may lead to abortion but to prevent abortion. I suggest that the present emphasis on the patient's right "to know"—to be given all the information necessary for decision-making—mandates that every woman

17. Y. C. Fletcher and M. I. Evans, "Maternal Bonding in Early Fetal Ultrasound Examinations," *New England Journal of Medicine*, vol. 308 (1983), pp. 392–393.

who requests an abortion be shown an ultrasound film of her developing fetus. Then let her decide. This approach will certainly decrease the number of abortions performed.

OTHER ISSUES RELATED TO ABORTION

A moratorium was imposed on fetal research for several years in the Unites States. Australia never imposed such a moratorium, however, and was thus able to advance ahead of the United States in the field of infertility management. Fetal research is essential for the study of infertility because it enables physicians to better understand the development of the fetus, especially in the early cleavage stages. There does not seem to be any halachic restriction on such research if it is limited to the use of spontaneously aborted fetuses.

A new area of halachic concern is the use of fetal tissue for transplantation in the treatment of patients with Alzheimer's or Parkinson's disease. American scientists have thus far been unable to reproduce the results reported by Mexican investigators who used autotransplants of adrenal gland tissue to treat patients with Parkinson's disease.[18] Some researchers have considered the use of fetal tissue for both Parkinson and Alzheimer patients. If this surgery proves effective, there would be a tremendous drive to procure fetal tissue. Some people might even consider intentional conception followed by willful abortion in order to provide fetal tissue for patients with these diseases. Ethical guidelines must be drawn up now, before the surgery is perfected.

Society is currently facing a number of other ethical dilemmas. There is, for example, a new "abortion pill" containing an antimetabolite and a prostaglandin compound;

---

18. A. N. Lieberman, "The Use of Adrenal Medullary and Fetal Grafts as a Treatment for Parkinson's Disease," *Journal of the American Medical Association*, vol. 263 (1990), pp. 565–570.

this may make abortion almost an at-home, over-the-counter kind of experience. Such a phenomenon presents a great threat to the sanctity of human life.

Another dilemma is that posed by pregnancy reduction. One of the great technical problems in in vitro fertilization is multiple pregnancy and the danger that such pregnancy entails for the mother as well as the viability of the fetuses. In Israel, physicians insert eight fertilized eggs at a time; in the United States they insert four; and in Australia they insert only two. The danger is that if four or more fetuses are successfully implanted, there is a possibility that none will survive unless some are aborted to allow the others to develop normally. There is also danger to the mother who is pregnant with multiple fetuses. At Mount Sinai Medical Center in New York, Dr. Richard Berkowitz performs pregnancy reduction as a "routine" procedure.[19] Halachically, this procedure requires careful analysis. Is this technique simply abortion with a euphonious name? Or is it indeed a permitted act because of the health threat to the mother or because of the questionable viability of the multiple embryos? If without reduction none will survive, then removal of some embryos to permit the others to develop normally cannot be viewed as the "taking of life."

This issue and the related issues of contraception and abortion that I have discussed here are extremely complex; for this reason, their halachic implications require more analysis than they can be given in this chapter.

---

19. R. L. Berkowitz, L. Lynch, V. Chitkara, et al., "Selective Reduction of Multifetal Pregnancies in the First Trimester," *New England Journal of Medicine*, vol. 318 (1988), pp. 1043–1057.

8

EUTHANASIA

Abraham S. Abraham, M.D.

*E*uthanasia, or mercy killing, is a term used today with wide implications, and in circumstances in which the suffering of the patient is not always the only deciding factor. In many instances, the suffering or burden caused to the patient's relatives or to the hospital or institution in which the patient is placed, or even to "society," are factors no less important. Recent legal decisions in the United States, in which the principles of "best interest" or "reasonable person" judgment were invoked—that is, what the court believed the patient would have wanted, had the patient been capable of self-determination—conferred on the court the combined status of prophet, prosecutor, judge, and God. The Nazis started by killing the old, the infirm, and the insane. Was that euthanasia? The contemporary Torah-observant physician, nurse, or medical assistant is exposed to ethical winds of today that are often derived from or even based entirely on what society or even the individual may accept as moral; but these "moral" judgments may be untouched by any understanding of, or even any need to consider, the will of the Creator of all life as taught to us by the Torah and our Sages. Nothing can replace the first-hand knowledge acquired from a discussion of a given situation with a recognized rabbinic authority, together with a serious attempt to study and understand the sources on which rabbinic decisions are based. Nevertheless, I will try to put forward in this chapter the halachic viewpoint as taught to me by my revered teachers—in particular, Rabbi Shlomo Zalman Auerbach.

HALACHIC PRINCIPLES

We have first to accept, and *then* to try to understand, three important and overriding principles:

1. The only situation in which one is allowed to kill another person is when the other is a potential murderer, and then only if such killing would result in the saving of one's own life or the life of another innocent individual. The Torah defines the potential murderer as a *rodef* (pursuer), who, by the act of pursuing, forfeits his life. Consequently, killing someone whose existence is not a threat to the life of another—be it a fetus, a newborn infant, or an adult—is murder.

2. One has no absolute ownership rights over one's own body.[1] The Almighty gave each of us a body and soul for a given time, and it is our duty when the time comes to return both to our Maker—just as one is responsible for, and obligated to look after, an article that is given for safe-keeping. There is no right to tamper with life unless for the purpose of preventing its destruction or loss.

3. Life, be it for 120 years or a split second, is itself of infinite value.[2] Thus, according to Rabbi Joseph Babad,

---

1. M. Feinstein, *Responsa Iggrot Moshe, Yoreh De'ah,* part 3, no. 140.

2. Y. Tukazinsky, *Gesher HaChayim,* part 1, chapter 2:2, note 3; S.Y. Zeven, *Halachah Urefuah,* vol. 2, ed. M. Hershler (Jerusalem, 1981), pp. 93–100. See also Y. Weinberg, *Responsa Seridei Aish,* part 2, no. 78.

known as Minchat Chinuch,[3] even if the prophet Elijah himself were to tell us that a given individual has only a few minutes to live, the Torah does not differentiate between one who kills a child who otherwise might live for many years and one who kills a 100-year-old person with only a limited life expectancy. Even if the victim were about to die anyway, the killer is a murderer because life has been curtailed—even if by only a second. Defining life in this way means that all of life, regardless of its quality and regardless of its duration, is of infinite value.

THE DYING PATIENT

This definition and its corollary may be difficult to accept when one is confronted with an individual who is suffering severe pain or mental agony because of a fatal disease and who prays for an end to life. It is well known that when Rabbi Yehudah Hanassi (Rabbi Judah the Prince, compiler of the Mishnah) was dying in pain, his maidservant, contrary to the wishes of his disciples, prayed for his death (*Ketubot* 104a). Based on this episode, Rabbi Nissim Gerondi, known as Ran,[4] rules that one may pray for the death of a suffering patient who is in such a condition. This decision is not ratified by many later authorities,[5] or by Rabbi Joseph Karo, author of *Shulchan Aruch*. However, both Rabbi Israel Lifschutz, known as Tiferet Yisrael,[6] and Rabbi Yechiel Michael Epstein,[7] author of *Aruch HaShulchan*, rule as Ran did. One must also remember that the prophets Elijah (I

---

3. *Minchat Chinuch*, Commandment no. 34.

4. Commentary *Ran* on Nedarim 40a.

5. E.Y. Waldenberg, *Responsa Tzitz Eliezer*, vol. 5, section *Ramat Rachel*, no. 5, and vol. 9, no. 47.

6. *Mishnah* commentary *Tiferet Yisrael* at the end of *Yoma*, *Yachin Uboaz*, no. 3.

7. *Aruch Hashulchan*, *Yoreh De'ah* 335: 3.

Kings 19:4) and Jonah (4:8) both prayed to die, as did Honi
Hama'agal (*Taanit* 23a).[8] However, neither Ran nor any of
the other sources quoted did more than advocate asking the
Almighty to release the patient from suffering.

Rabbi Moshe Feinstein[9] writes that it is certainly forbidden to try to prolong the life of a dying person if this
effort would result in additional pain and suffering. But to
shorten life, even a life of agony and suffering, is, in his view,
forbidden. If one does so—albeit for reasons of compassion
and even at the request of the patient—one is a murderer and
punishable by death.

It is taken for granted that a patient in pain should be
treated with any and as much pain-relieving medication as is
necessary. Under no circumstances, however, must such
medication be administered in order to *shorten* life.[10]

This world is but a corridor to the world to come. It is
not for us to question the ways of the Almighty. The enigma
of the sufferings of the righteous and the bliss of the wicked
remains for us unanswerable.[11]

I recently treated a patient with end-stage emphysema.
This 65-year-old man, who was hypoxic (oxygen-deficient)
even while being given eight liters of oxygen per minute,
fought for every breath. He managed to painfully gasp out
his request that I inject "something to make him sleep
forever." He was tired of suffering, tired of burdening his

---

8. See also the story of Rabbi Yochanan's death (*Baba Metzia* 84a, at the end
of the page) and the examples related in the Jerusalem Talmud (*Yerushalmi,
Shabbat* 19:2, at the end of the page); and the collection of biblical commentaries
known as *Yalkut Shimoni* (on *Parshat Ekev*, no. 871; and Proverbs, no. 943).

9. *Responsa Iggrot Moshe, Yoreh De'ah* 2:174.

10. A.S. Abraham, *Nishmat Avraham, Yoreh De'ah* 339:4, at the end, quoted in
the name of Rabbi Shlomo Zalman Auerbach. See also Rabbi Avigdor Nebenzahl
in *Assia*, vol. 7 (May 1980), pp. 39–41.

11. See also the Talmud (*Menachot* 29b and *Berachot* 61b) with regard to Rabbi
Akiva's death, and Maimonides' famous code (*Mishneh Torah, Hilchot Sotah*
3:20).

wife and family, and tired of the supreme effort of breathing. Two years previously he had been admitted to our respiratory intensive care unit (ICU) with pneumonia, and had been intubated there for many days. At the time he had written, "Please let me die"; the note was still in his file. This patient's mental and physical pain was truly an agonizing, heartbreaking thing to witness. One of our conversations, during rounds one day and in the presence of the patient's wife, left few dry eyes among those in attendance. "What have the last two years been like before your admission to the ICU?" I asked him now.

"A living death, worth nothing," he replied.

"Do you have any grandchildren?" I asked.

"Yes, four."

"Do they visit you?"

"Yes, often," he said and his face lit up.

"And do you enjoy them?" I asked.

"What a question!" he said. "Every minute is Heaven!"

"Worth living for?" I asked. There was no answer.

"Were these two years wasted?" Silence.

Halachah is quite clear and categoric on this point. Under no circumstances may the active killing of a patient be justified or condoned. No matter what, it is an act of murder. The fact that the patient pleads for this to be done does not alter the perpetrator's ultimate responsibility for committing murder, one of the three cardinal sins of Judaism which can never be set aside.

Except for murder, idolatry, and forbidden sexual relations such as incest, one is obligated to set aside all Sabbath and other biblical and rabbinic rulings by performing what are otherwise Torah-prohibited acts if this is necessary to save life. Therefore, writes Rabbi Auerbach,[12] although it is obvious to all that the life of a paralyzed person is not a

---

12. *Halachah Urefuah*, vol. 3, ed. M. Hershler (Jerusalem, 1983), p. 60.

valuable life according to our simplistic idea, and in spite of
the very real suffering of the patient and family, we are
nevertheless commanded to do everything in our power to
prolong life. If such a person takes sick, it is our duty to do
everything we can to save his life, even by setting aside the
Sabbath. We have no yardstick by which to measure the
worth and importance of a human life, not even in terms of
the Torah it will learn and the commandments (*mitzvot*) it
will keep. One must set aside the Sabbath even for one who
is old and sick, one who may be socially unacceptable
because of a revolting external disease, or one who may be
mentally retarded and incapable of fulfilling any commandment. This approach is true even if the patient is a severe
burden and source of suffering to members of the family,
who are themselves thereby prevented from studying Torah
and performing precepts, and even if the patient, in addition
to causing others great suffering, imposes a severe financial
strain on his family. Moreover, if the patient is suffering so
much that it is a meritorious act to pray for his death (as
ruled by Ran, noted earlier), nevertheless, while one prays to
the Almighty that the patient die, one must simultaneously
do everything in one's power to save the patient, even if so
doing requires that the Sabbath be repeatedly set aside (to be
discussed later in the chapter).

PASSIVE EUTHANASIA

The problem becomes more complicated when one considers passive euthanasia. "Allowing someone to die" can run a
wide spectrum, from withholding treatment or life-saving
procedures at one extreme to withholding food and drink at
the other. Withholding treatment may include not only the
withholding of antibiotics for infection but also the withholding of life-sustaining substances such as insulin, blood,
or oxygen. Which, if any, of these approaches is permitted?

The underlying principle of passive euthanasia—the removal of causes that prevent the death of the dying patient—is well documented. The case of Rabbi Chanina ben Teradion,[13] who agreed to have the soaking cotton wool removed from around his chest so that his death by burning would not be prolonged, is well known. Rabbi Moshe Isserles,[14] in his glossary on the *Shulchan Aruch*, cites examples of what is permitted in order to remove any hindrance to the departure of the soul (i.e., death). As mentioned earlier, Ran permits one to pray for a patient's death. The inhabitants of the legendary city of Luz, where no one ever died, went outside the city wall when they tired of life (*Sotah* 46b). (This talmudic statement is at first sight difficult to explain because it describes a positive act in which the person walked outside the city walls in order to die. In actuality, this act led only, *indirectly* to death by "natural causes." Also, the Talmud merely states what the citizens of Luz did, without discussing the right or wrong of their actions.)

The question, therefore, is to what extent and under which circumstances one may desist from treating a dying patient. It is obvious from what Rabbi Auerbach writes that a patient with Alzheimer's disease or with severe cerebral damage, whatever the cause, is still a human being in the fullest sense of the word, and must be considered as such in the context of active euthanasia. Furthermore, according to his view,[15] any procedure needed to nourish or sustain the patient must be carried out, even if this can be done only by artificial means. Thus, the patient must be given food and drink even if this may be possible only by means of a nasogastric feeding tube or feeding jejunostomy, or by total

---

13. Abodah Zarah 18a; see also *Responsa Iggrot Moshe, Yoreh De'ah*, part 2, no. 174:3; and *Choshen Mishpat*, part 2, no. 73:3, and no. 74:2.

14. M. Isserles, J. Karo's *Shulchan Aruch, Yoreh De'ah* 339:1.

15. *Nishmat Avraham, Yoreh De'ah 339:4.*

parenteral nutrition—exactly as one would do for any other patient who needed such treatment and who had a full chance of recovery. Similarly, required daily insulin injections must be given, just as oxygen and blood must be given when necessary. I was recently involved in the case of a 68-year-old woman who had been on a hemodialysis program for some eighteen months, and who suffered a major intracerebral hemorrhage and cardiac arrest. She was intubated and resuscitated by her medical attendants. I asked Rabbi Auerbach whether dialysis should be continued on such a deeply comatose, respirator-dependent patient. His answer was an unqualified yes; since she was already on such a program, this was for her a "normal" procedure.

Many years ago a 63-year-old man with end-stage diabetic nephropathy, neuropathy, cardiomyopathy, and retinopathy was admitted to my care. This blind man, who had had a below-knee amputation for gangrene two years earlier, was admitted with sepsis, congestive cardiac failure, and moist gangrene of the other leg. The chance of his living for more than a few days without surgical intervention was obviously nil, but in view of his extremely poor general condition, the surgeons determined that if they were to proceed with the surgery he would have little chance of leaving the operating room alive. The man himself refused surgery and wished to be left to die. Rabbi Auerbach decided that we should not insist on the operation, since this would not be curative of the underlying condition, was highly risky, and would only add to the patient's physical and mental suffering; in addition, the patient himself did not want the operation. He died a few days later.

Rabbi Feinstein[16] also writes that if there is no known treatment available for the patient, and there are no means by which to relieve suffering, and all that can be done is to

---

16. *Iggrot Moshe, Choshen Mishpat*, part 2, nos. 72, 75.

prolong a life of agony for a short while, one should not do so but should provide only supportive care and allow nature to take its course.

TREATMENT OF THE TERMINALLY ILL

A general approach to the problem can therefore be summarized as follows:

1. All patients must be given food, drink, oxygen, and other normally accepted life-sustaining measures, even if such treatment must be given in an unusual manner.

2. A patient with a chronic, incapacitating, but not terminal illness (i.e., one that is not expected to result in a speedy death) must be treated exactly as any other patient would be, and full resuscitative measures must be carried out if required, even if they are likely to prolong life for only a short while.

3. A terminally ill patient who is close to death must be treated as any other patient would be in terms of daily sustenance and accepted medical care. However, if the patient is in cardiac or respiratory arrest or both, or develops a complication that requires a major treatment procedure that will *add* to the suffering, then the following guidelines should be observed:

(a) If the arrest is as expected in the natural course of the terminal illness, one need not resuscitate, and indeed it may be wrong to do so. In addition, desperate major measures to prolong the final inevitable death process, measures which will add further agony and suffering, should not be taken.

(b) If, however, the arrest arises unexpectedly, from a cause unrelated to the underlying disease, or if a complication develops that is unconnected to the disease, full treatment must be given as for any other patient unless this will cause further suffering to the patient over and above that caused by his original disease.

Thus, all patients must be given normal sustenance and treatment. The majority of patients should be treated as symptoms indicate, even by major medical or surgical intervention, including resuscitation. There is a small minority of patients (described in 3a above) for whom major intervention and resuscitation are not appropriate.

Obviously, no two patients and no two cases are alike. Therefore it cannot be stated too strongly that no decision relating to life and death should be made without prior consultation with a recognized rabbinic authority. Nothing is more final than murder.

I must at this point add something that I have found to be easily forgotten or overlooked. Let us suppose that the patient is suffering from a terminal illness, is expected to die in a few hours or days (group 3a again), and is one for whom the medical profession has nothing further to offer. Such a patient should be made as comfortable as possible and treated with a maximum of tender loving care; such treatment may include the administration of morphine or its equivalent to relieve pain, but not for the purpose of ending life. Once such a stage has been reached, based on the realization that nothing of further value can be done, a second order must be issued to all involved in the patient's care: No more tests or examinations! Is there any point to routine pulse, temperature, or blood pressure recordings, or especially the withdrawal of blood for testing purposes, once the stage of illness has been reached when nothing further of value can be done regardless of any change in the patient's condition? Certainly, the performance of such an act on the Sabbath would be a pointless desecration. Finally, when close to death, the patient should not be moved or touched except for his own comfort or benefit.[17]

TREATMENT OF HANDICAPPED NEWBORNS

What about the baby born with an untreatable, rapidly fatal heart defect? Or the anencephalic baby? Are they to be considered "alive," and therefore to have everything necessary to keep them alive done for them even on the Sabbath? Or are they to be considered already "dead" (since we know that they will not live for thirty days), meaning not only that nothing must be done for them on the Sabbath (even if this involves a rabbinic prohibition only) but also that organs may be removed from them for transplantation even in the presence of spontaneous respiration and heartbeat? The Talmud (*Shabbat* 135a) states that under certain circumstances a baby born in the eighth month of gestation is likened to a stone (i.e., nonviable) and may not be moved (on the Sabbath), but the mother may lean over him so that he may suckle, because of the danger. Rashi explains that "the danger" refers to the mother, since an excess of milk may lead to illness. Thus, at first reading, it appears that a baby born following eight months of gestation and believed unable to live for thirty days was considered in the Talmud to be already "dead." It would then be a desecration even of rabbinic ordinances to feed such a child on the Sabbath. However, Rabbi Meir Abulafia, known as Yad Ramah,[18] and Rashi (*Yebamot* 80b) both explain "the danger" as being applicable to either the baby or the mother. Therefore, Rabbi Auerbach explains that the Talmud refers to a case in which (1) the baby lies motionless and unresponding "like a stone," and (2) it was born prematurely; only in such a case

---

17. *Shulchan Aruch, Yoreh De'ah* 339:1.
18. Commentary *Yad Ramah* on *Baba Bathra* 10a.

is it prohibited to desecrate the Sabbath for the baby even if by so doing one might prolong "transient life" by a few hours or days, since we are dealing with a baby who will *definitely* die within thirty days. However, if the baby moves and responds to stimuli it should be treated as normal, even if it is certain that it will live for only a few days, and even if it means desecrating the Sabbath. This rule applies all the more if the baby was born at term.

The anencephalic child (complete or incomplete) will certainly die within thirty days after birth. More than 95 percent of such babies die within seventy-two hours. However, an anencephalic newborn moves its limbs, makes crying noises, and sucks, all of which are spinal reflexes; no cerebrum is present. Rabbi Yitzchak Zilberstein[19] states that it is permissible to abort such a fetus because halachically it is not considered alive but is considered within the category of a *nevelah* (corpse). His ruling is based on the Talmud (*Niddah* 24a) and on Maimonides,[20] where it is stated that such a fetus, when born, does not render the mother ritually unclean. What, then, is its status once born? Rabbi Abraham Zvi Eisenstadt, known as Pitchei Teshuvah,[21] quotes the ruling of Rabbi Eleazar Fleckeles, author of *Responsa Tshuvah MeAhavah*, who ruled that the fact that a child does not render the mother ritually unclean as a result of its birth does not mean that one has the right to kill it. This would be tantamount to murder, even if the death is brought about passively, such as by starvation. In fact, death by starvation would be worse, for the sin of cruelty would be added to the sin of murder. Rabbi Auerbach[22] concurs with this ruling of *Tshuvah MeAhavah*. He states that even though it would probably be permissible to *abort* such a fetus, once it is born

---

19. In a lecture series he presented to a group of physicians.
20. *Mishneh Torah, Hilchot Issurei Biyah* 10:11.
21. Commentary *Pitchei Teshuvah* on *Shulchan Aruch, Yoreh De'ah* 194:5.
22. Personal communication.

it may not be killed, and one is obligated to desecrate the Sabbath on its behalf, if necessary, especially if it was born at term. If such a baby stopped breathing or suffered cardiac arrest, however, resuscitation need not be carried out.

CONCLUSIONS

We should approach the problems of life and death with humility, with the realization of our fallibility and lack of absolute knowledge, with complete acceptance of the tenets of the Torah *as expounded by our Sages*, with the readiness to listen to and put into practice what *they* tell us, and with the willingness to control our emotions—even those of pity and compassion—within the boundaries set by the Torah. Only thus can we again achieve the heights we all reached at Mount Sinai when, as one, we vowed "*Naase veNishma*" (We will do and we will learn).

It behooves us all to read and read again what Maimonides wrote in his Code:[23]

It is fitting to give thought to the Laws of our Holy Torah and to delve into their meanings to the best of one's ability. And, if one does not find a logical reason for or does not understand something, it must not then become unimportant in one's eyes . . . One must not attempt to reach the understanding of the Almighty since this will surely lead to harm; neither must one think of the Torah with the same human logic with which one faces one's daily problems. Come and see how strict the Torah is with the Laws of wrongful use of things that were sanctified. If sticks and stones, dust and ashes, once a human being has dedicated them even by word-of-mouth only, become truly sanctified,

---

23. *Mishneh Torah, Hilchot Meilah* 8:8.

and one who desecrates such sanctity is held guilty, and is required to bring a sacrificial offering, even if the act were unintentional, then how much more so that the commandments that were given to us by the Almighty may not be transgressed and belittled, just because we do not fully understand their meaning.

In the modern world of fast-moving technological medicine in which we live, where today's taboo is tomorrow's routine, and where yesterday's unthinkable becomes today's debatable and then tomorrow's unexceptional, we, as religious and believing Jews, must strengthen and reaffirm our faith in the Almighty and His Torah as the ultimate and indeed the only way to lead and shape every part of our lives and even our very thoughts. We must take this approach even if it forces us to reach the unpalatable realization and conclusion that we are fallible in our logic and understanding.

Against your will do you live, and against your will do you die, and against your will are you destined to give account and reckoning before the Supreme King of kings, the Holy One, blessed be He. [*Abot* 4:29]

9

THE DEFINITION OF DEATH

Abraham Steinberg, M.D.

It is not my intent in this chapter to render halachic judgment on the definition of death. This task is certainly beyond my capability. It is also not for me to speak on behalf of the great luminaries of the Torah. I present the following thoughts in all humility and reverence. My intent is to assist the *poskim* (rabbinic decisors) in determining Halachah in this matter. Rendering judgment on matters of life and death requires accurate and relevant medical facts. With a proper understanding of the facts and the underlying data, the rabbi can adjudicate in the spirit and letter of the law, an approach used in all factual–scientific endeavors. This has always been so.[1] As a neurologist, I will attempt in this chapter to present clearly and concisely the scientific data relevant to the determination of the time of death. The seemingly decisive language used in this chapter should not be interpreted as a final adjudication in Jewish law. Rather, I present a halachic approach and interpretation for consideration by the *poskim* of our generation.

---

1. S. Z. Auerbach, Introduction to *Me'orey Aish* (Jerusalem: Beth Medrash Moriah, 1980).

The question before us deals with the laws relating to the preservation of life. It is incumbent upon whomever can provide clarification of the halachic implications of a subject to do so. This chapter, therefore, represents merely "a student deliberating before his teachers." For more than a decade I have studied the issue of determining the moment of death, and have published several articles on various aspects of the subject in which I summarized the various rabbinic opinions.[2] In this chapter, following renewed and extensive study of halachic sources, I have come to conclusions different from those I published in the past. However, these conclusions do not dictate Halachah; rather, they represent suggestions for further analysis and discussion of the difficult questions of the Halachic definition of death.

GENERAL CONSIDERATIONS

The halachic definition of death has a direct bearing upon the issue of the preservation of life of potential organ recipients. If it is halachically determined that death does not occur until the cessation of cardiac activity, removing a heart for transplantation while it is still beating is tantamount to murder of the donor, no different than the killing of the terminally ill.[3] On the other hand, if death is halachically determined by brain death, abstaining from taking the donor's heart for transplantation until the heart stops will cause the death of the potential recipient, whose continued life depends on receiving a heart transplant. A halachically binding definition of death is essential because the lives of potential organ recipients are at stake.

---

2. A. Steinberg, *Noam*, vol. 19 (1977), pp. 210–238; *Harefuah*, vol. 98 (1980), pp. 412–414; *Sefer Assia*, vol. 3 (Jerusalem: Rubin Mass, 1982), pp. 393–432.

3. M. Maimonides, *Mishneh Torah, Hilchot Rotze'ach Ushemirat Hanefesh* 2:7–8; Y. Z. Meklenberg, *Haketav Vehakabalah*, Genesis 9:5.

The tremendous medical and technological advances of recent years include the availability of sophisticated resuscitation equipment that can artificially prolong a person's respiration, resulting in extended prolongation of the heart's function. This technology makes for a separation in time between the classic signs of death (i.e., between the lack of respiration and the absence of heartbeat). Parallel technical advances have been made in surgical techniques and immunology that enable us to retard or prevent rejection of transplanted organs. As a result, heart and other organ transplants are performed today as routinely as other major surgical procedures. At large medical centers, the current survival rate after heart transplants is 70 to 80 percent at one year and 55 to 65 percent at five years following the procedure.

The medical–scientific determination of brain death today, provided that this definition of death is halachically valid, is more reliable than the classical method for determining death (i.e., absence of spontaneous respiration and heartbeat).

The heart is vital to life. Life is not possible in its absence. The crucial issue, however, is the following: Is cessation of the heart's activity an integral and necessary part of the halachic definition of death? The liver, the pancreas, the kidneys, the bone marrow, and other body organs are all essential to life, but none is used as a criterion in defining death. Why is the heart different?

From the metaphysical standpoint, the heart may be the source of the soul, emotion, wisdom, feeling, will, and so on. The Sages differ in their opinions on this issue. The Midrash[4] states: "Where is the source of wisdom? . . . Rabbi Eliezer says in the head, and Rabbi Joshua says in the heart." Rabbi Bachya ben Asher,[5] known as Rabbenu Bechayei, says: "And the brain—the sanctuary of the spiri-

---

4. Proverbs *Rabbah* 1.
5. *Chovot Halevavot, Shaar Habechinah.*

tual powers and the fountain from which feelings spring."
The famous *Tanya*, authored by Rabbi Shneur Zalman of
Liadi,[6] states: "The sanctuary of the divine soul is in the brain
lodged in the head and from there spreads to all the organs."
Finally, in the words of Rabbi Menachem Azaria of Pano:[7]
"And from there the breath went straight to the brain, the
sanctuary of the intelligence and called by our Sages the
soul."

Clearly the Sages were divided in their opinions as to
the seat of the soul; some, but not all, attribute it to the heart.
This metaphysical discussion, however, is not relevant to the
halachic definition of death, which must be based on scientific and purely halachic considerations.

In the Talmud, and for early post-talmudic decisors
(*rishonim*), absence of spontaneous *respiration* is the only
significant, reliable sign of death. Indeed, absence of respiration is not in itself viewed as death, but rather as a sign of
dysfunction of a more basic organ that controls the breathing
mechanism and whose nonfunction defines the moment of
death. Which is that organ? How is it determined? The two
possibilities are the heart and the brain; this question will be
discussed in these pages.

Biological death is a continuous process. Various cells
and organs die or cease to function at different times,
according to their relative sensitivity to lack of oxygen,
blood, and other vital elements. Determination of a specific
moment in this process is based on social, judicial—and, for
observant Jews, halachic—criteria. Death is not determined
only after signs of decay are apparent, which is the biological
criterion for absolute death of all body cells. Rather, death is
determined to occur at an earlier stage, when halachically
accepted and defined signs are apparent even though, from a
biological standpoint, there are still living cells and organs in
the body.

---

6. *Tanya*, chapter 9.
7. *Ma'amar Hanefesh*, chapter 3.

The whole issue of brain death is solely concerned with a person who is devoid of autonomous respiration and is connected to a respirator. Continued vitality of the various organs of such a person, including the heart, depends on artificial respiration. Is a person in whom it can be medically proved that autonomous respiration will never resume considered halachically alive or dead, even if the heart is still beating?

Our discussion here does not deal with the public aspects of organ transplantation under conditions of limited resources. How should a transplant recipient be chosen, among the many waiting for this treatment, when there are not enough organs for all? Can we depend on physicians to base their choice of an organ recipient on halachic grounds? Can we rely on physicians to adhere to the halachic definition of the moment of death? These are serious and controversial questions that each deserve a separate hearing, based on defined guidelines and principles. They are not our primary concern in this chapter.

The halachic problems and considerations for organ donors are different from those for recipients, and not dependent one on the other. In regard to the donor, the central issue is the determination of the moment of death; a successful heart or liver transplant requires removing these organs from the donor while the heart is still beating. From the point of view of the recipient, the central question is whether these procedures are still experimental or whether the current excellent survival rates justify considering them as standard treatments. Additional halachic problems will be considered later in this chapter.

HISTORICAL BACKGROUND

In 1772, the Duke of Mecklenburg issued an edict prohibiting early burial of the dead in this former duchy in eastern

Germany, and required that there be an interim period of
three days between clinical death and burial. Before burial,
the body of the deceased had to exhibit "death spots" and
signs of the body's decay. The intent was to prevent the
burying of people who had been mistakenly diagnosed as
dead. Fears of the possibility of "false" deaths were so
rampant in Mecklenburg in the eighteenth century that the
dead were buried in a special coffin built with an air vent and
a bell that could be heard above ground should the deceased
come to life.

The duke's edict aroused strong halachic objections
among the Jews of that period. The Enlightened—led by
Moses Mendelssohn—defended the duke's order. Mendelssohn published an article in which he tried to prove that
this command was halachically correct.[8] In a response to
the article, Rabbi Yaakov Emden[9] refuted all of Mendelssohn's evidence. During that period, however, many
states prohibited the prompt burial of the deceased, and
this edict was reluctantly followed by the Jews. Rabbi
Moshe Schreiber,[10] known as Chatam Sofer, wrote: "It
seems to me that, because of the royal edict, we became
accustomed to delaying burial, [so] Jews mistakenly think
that this custom derives from the Law of the Torah." He
again refuted Mendelssohn's evidence and ruled that burial
must take place as soon as possible after death has been
determined.

Delaying the burial of the dead is prohibited by biblical
law. Preparation for burial should start within an hour of the
clinical determination of death.[11] In setting a time for burial,
one need not take into account the extremely rare occurrence

---

8. *Bikurei Ha'Itim* (1823), pp. 82 ff.
9. *Bikurei Ha'Itim* (1824), pp. 229–232.
10. *Responsa Chatam Sofer, Yoreh De'ah*. no. 338.
11. Y. M. Tukazinsky, *Gesher HaChayim*, part 1, chapter 1; S. Gagin, *Responsa Yismach Lev, Yoreh De'ah*, no. 9.

of a mistake in the determination of death.[12] Rabbi Chaim Yosef David Azulai wrote: "If one in several tens of thousands of buried persons turns out later to be alive, we should not see this as a basis for a prohibition [against prompt burial], for that was decreed upon him . . . if they erred in the signs [of death], this is Divine Will, and there is no prohibition whatsoever; all that was done was by the Law of the Torah."[13]

Until recently, death was medically defined as the cessation of spontaneous respiration and cardiac activity. About thirty years ago the concept of brain death was introduced. An integral part of the definition of brain death in a patient attached to a respirator is the lack of spontaneous respiration even while the heart continues to function. Prior to the development of sophisticated means of resuscitation it was impossible, in a person whose breathing had stopped because of brain damage, for the heart to continue beating for more than a few minutes. Today, the heart of such a person can continue to beat for hours and even days if respiration is artifically maintained.

Three conditions must exist to accurately determine brain death:

1. The entire brain, including the brainstem, has ceased to function, as evidenced by specific clinical and laboratory tests.
2. The patient's disease is known, is incurable, and does not derive from factors that can be treated.
3. Brain death is final and irreversible; that is, all tests show total brain death after a period of several hours (the number varies, in accordance with different opinions) have passed.

---

12. *Semachot* 8:1; Z. H. Chayes, *Responsa Maharitz Chayes*, no. 52; S. M. Schwadron, *Responsa Maharsham*, part 6, no. 91.
13. *Responsa Chayim Sha'al*, part 2, no. 25.

If a transplant of one of the patient's organs is anticipated, brain death is determined by members of the medical staff not taking part in the transplant, to assure utmost objectivity.

MEDICAL–SCIENTIFIC BACKGROUND

The brain consists of several parts. The two main parts are (1) the cerebrum, or upper brain, which controls consciousness, thought, understanding, memory, feeling, and voluntary movement; and (2) the brainstem, which controls the transmission to and from the rest of the body of all the functions of the cerebrum. The brainstem also controls vital functions such as swallowing, sleep and waking cycles, and, most important, respiration and cardiac activity.

There is indeed a major difference between the brainstem's supervision of respiration and its supervision of the heart, in that natural respiration is totally and singularly dependent on the sustained activity of the brainstem. The lungs are incapable of carrying out respiration unless activated by the respiratory center, located in the brainstem. The purpose of respiration is the exchange of the gases vital to life—inhalation of oxygen and exhalation of carbon dioxide.

Although the heart's activity is also regulated by the brainstem, the heart has, in addition, an autonomous system in the form of a natural pacemaker. As long as the heart is adequately supplied with oxygen, blood, and nutrients, it can continue to beat for several minutes to several days even outside the body. The autonomous activity of the heart is similar to the severed tail of a lizard, as described by Maimonides: "When the power of movement is no longer disseminated throughout the body's organs from one source and beginning."[14] These autonomous movements are reflex-

---

14. *Mishnah* commentary, *Oholot* 1:16.

ive and are not derived from the central nervous system. Such movements are not a sign of life but a local reflex action which has no vital significance.

When the cerebrum ceases to function, a person lies motionless in bed and is no longer aware of his surroundings. Yet the vital life functions, including autonomous respiration (without the aid of a respirator), regular heart function, digestion, and sleep and wake cycles, continue in an orderly manner. This condition, known as the persistent vegetative state, represents not brain death but a state of life with altered consciousness. In contrast, when the brainstem ceases to function, vital life activities—including respiration—also cease. Without an artificial respirator, all other organs also cease to function. This state constitutes total brain death and, therefore, organismal death.

In summary, the sequence of natural death starts with total brain death, which results in cessation of spontaneous respiration, followed by cardiac death. Biologically, there is a direct link between the brainstem and natural respiration, but there is no direct link between respiration and the heart. Cardiac arrest rapidly causes brain death because it results in a lack of blood supply to the brain, which leads to termination of breathing. Similarly, cessation of liver and kidney function eventually results in brain death; the inability of the liver to produce essential materials and the inability of the kidney to excrete poisons lead to cessation of spontaneous respiration. In this respect the heart is no different from any other vital organ.

Until recently, medicine could do little to intervene in the process, and the three classic death signs—death of the brain, cessation of respiration, and cessation of heartbeat—occurred within minutes of each other. Today, an artificial respirator can help the patient breathe even if the brainstem is no longer functional. Such artificial respiration permits other body organs, including the heart, to continue to function. The heart can thus continue to provide blood to the body by means of its internal control system. Because autonomous breathing is not possible when the brainstem has completely stopped functioning, as has been described, such a patient is completely dependent on mechanical artificial respiration. The heart and other organs, such as the liver and kidneys, can continue to function for a certain period of time as long as artificial respiration is continued. Withdrawal of the respirator machine causes cessation of the heartbeat and gradually leads to the termination of activity of other organs, each according to its sensitivity to lack of oxygen and blood supply.

It is possible today to accurately diagnose brain death, including brainstem death, by means of clinical examination and auxiliary tests. Such tests include apnea tests; cerebral blood flow studies, such as radioisotope studies, Doppler tests, and cerebral arteriograms; and electrophysiological examinations. (The electroencephalogram is insufficient to determine total brain death.) One or more of these tests should be performed and then repeated six to twelve hours later to ensure the finality and irreversibility of brainstem death. Conditions that mimic brain death, such as hypothermia or narcotic overdose, must be ruled out. If the tests indicate total and absolute dysfunction of the entire brain including the brainstem, then this is absolute proof that brain death is final and irreversible and there is no possibility that autonomous respiration will begin anew. Such a diagnosis of brain death requires proficiency, expertise, and adequate auxiliary tests. Until these studies have been completed, the patient is not considered dead, but rather doubtfully alive. On the other hand, following the absolute determination of death he is considered retroactively dead, from the first moment at which the tests indicated a lack of autonomous respiration.

The halachic definition of death requires ascertainment that spontaneous respiration has ceased completely and irreversibly. This point is biologically indicated by the absolute cessation of the activity of the entire brain, including that of the brainstem. Indeed, what is imperative is proof of final and irreversible absence of brain activity, rather than anatomical damage to all parts of the brain, for even in the classic method of determining death—absence of cardiac and respiratory activity—no proof of damage to the heart muscle is required; rather, only the irreversible absence of the heart's activity must be demonstrated.

HALACHIC CONSIDERATIONS

Classic Jewish Sources

The main talmudic text dealing with the question of the determination of the moment of death is the following: "If a building collapses on a person [on the Sabbath] . . . they [may] dig to remove the rubble from him [to try to save his life] . . . but if he is dead, they leave him there [until after the Sabbath]. How far does one check [to determine whether or not he is dead]? Until his nostrils; and some say, Until his heart" (*Yoma* 85a). This ruling to check the nostrils to determine life or death is codified in Jewish law.[15] The Talmud continues: "Rabbi Pappa said that the disagreement is when one examines from below to above, but [when] from above to below—since he examined him until his nostrils—he need [examine] no more" (*Yoma* 85a). This ruling is explicitly stated by Rabbi Joseph Karo in his *Shulchan Aruch*.[16]

Maimonides states: "And when one comes to his nos-

---

15. M. Maimonides, *Mishneh Torah, Hilchot Shabbat* 2:19; and J. Karo, *Shulchan Aruch, Orach Chayim* 329:4.

16. *Orach Chayim* 329:4. See also M. Feinstein, *Responsa Iggrot Moshe, Yoreh De'ah* 2:146, who states that Maimonides certainly holds that Halachah follows the opinion of Rav Pappa.

trils and does not find any breath in him, then one may not dig any more, since he is undoubtedly dead."[17] Rabbi Shlomo ben Yitzchak,[18] known as Rashi, similarly writes: "And if there is no vitality in his nostrils in that one does not find any wind [i.e., breath], he is undoubtedly dead, and [if it is on the Sabbath] one leaves him." Rashi and Maimonides take pains to stress that in the absence of breathing the person is *undoubtedly dead*; one must leave him, and it is prohibited to dig any further on the Sabbath, even though any doubt regarding the *saving* of life overrides the Sabbath. Neither Rashi nor Maimonides, while interpreting the opinion that considers the sign of absent respiration from the nostrils as halachically valid, mentions the heart as a criterion for determining death.

The talmudic text thus contains a disagreement as to which organ's cessation determines the fact of death. According to one opinion, death is determined by observing the nostrils (i.e., respiration), and according to the other, by listening for the heartbeat. This latter version, however, is cited by only a very few talmudic commentators.[19] However, the Jerusalem Talmud (*Yerushalmi Yoma* 8e) and most early talmudic commentators (*rishonim*) substitute the word *navel* for *heart*.[20] Rabbi Moses ben Simon Margoliot, known as Penei Moshe, explains that even the rabbis who adopt the textual reading of "navel" are of the opinion that breathing is the decisive sign, and that the navel provides a sign similar to that of the nostrils.[21] The examination of the navel refers to diaphragmatic breathing,[22] which is perceived near the na-

17. Commentary on the *Mishnah, Yoma*, loc. cit.

18. Rashi's commentary on *Yoma* 85a, caption *Ad Chotemo*.

19. Ibid., and M. Meiri, Commentary *Meiri* on *Yoma* 85a.

20. Rabbeinu Chananel, Rif (Rabbeinu Isaac ben Jacob Alfasi), Rabbeinu Jonathan of Lunel, Rivevan (Rabbi Judah ben Benjamin haRofe), and Rosh (Rabbeinu Asher) on *Yoma* 85a, and *Bet Yosef* on *Tur, Orach Chayim,* no. 329.

21. Commentary on *Yerushalmi Yoma* 8e.

22. A. Steinberg, *Sefer Assia*, vol. 3 (Jerusalem: Rubin Mass, 1983), p. 405.

vel. Nonetheless, even the version "until his heart" is not in accordance with the final halachic ruling, which is "until his nostrils." Furthermore, according to the opinion of Rav Pappa, and to Halachah, there is no disagreement over what is to be done when the rescuer first encounters the victim's head in the rubble of the collapsed building; he is to remove the rubble until the victim's nostrils are visible. If the *heart* is decisive in determining the moment of death, why did the talmudic Sages not obligate the rescuer to remove rubble until the heart? And how did Maimonides determine that if there is no breath in the nostrils, he is "undoubtedly" dead?

The literal reading of the key talmudic text and the comments of the *rishonim* clearly imply that the vital sign distinguishing between life and death is breathing, and not the beating of the heart. Rabbi Moshe Schreiber similarly writes: "For everything is dependent upon the breath of the nose, as is explained in *Yoma* 85a; and in the ruling in Maimonides and the *Tur Shulchan Aruch*."[23] Rabbi Moshe Feinstein also states: "It is explicitly stated in the Gemara, *Yoma* 85a, . . . and similarly there is a ruling in Maimonides . . . and in the *Shulchan Aruch* . . . that [the ruling that] if they did not sense any vitality, he is legally dead, refers to the examination of breathing . . . and if they see that he is not breathing, this is the sign of death upon which we can rely, and there is no need to ponder this; see the [writings of] the Chatam Sofer. . . ."[24] These rabbinic decisors (*poskim*) make no mention of the heart in reference to the text in Yoma, nor do they mention pulses in the arteries or temples, as some authorities suggest in their interpretations of this talmudic text. Thus, the heart has no halachic status in the definition of the moment of death, and it is wrong to append to the text in *Yoma* any conditions,

---

23. M. Schreiber, *Responsa Chatam Sofer, Yoreh De'ah*, no. 338, entry *Ve-Nehezi*.

24. M. Feinstein, *Responsa Iggrot Moshe, Yoreh De'ah*, 3:132.

casuistry, and hairsplitting that are not there. Some contemporary rabbis posit that a distinction should be made between the case in *Yoma*, which speaks of a person covered by
debris, and regular death, in which case the heart must be
checked. This approach was rejected by the Chatam Sofer,
who wondered how such a distinction could be made, since
the biblical expression "breath of the spirit of life" (Genesis
7:22) does not refer to debris.[25]

The emphasis of the Talmud in *Yoma* that, regarding the
saving of life, the main sign of vitality is in the nose clearly
implies that the definition of life and death on the basis of
breathing is an essential matter of principle, and not a mere
"technical" matter. Furthermore, there are cases in which a
person's heart continues to beat, but the person nevertheless
is halachically regarded as dead. Maimonides rules: "If his
neck is broken, and most of the flesh with it, or he is torn
like a fish from his back, or his head was cut off, or he is
divided into two parts in his stomach—this situation imparts
impurity [as a corpse], even though one of his limbs still
flutters."[26] Although the heart still beats, this mortally
wounded person is regarded as having died immediately.
Thus, the activity of the heart per se does not necessarily
constitute a sign of life. Indeed, there is no allusion in the
entire Talmud to the heart as an essential factor in the determination of the moment of death, except for the aforementioned version by a minority of *rishonim*. This opinion,
however, does not constitute the final Halachah. On the
contrary, throughout Jewish writings, breathing is discussed
as the determinant of the transition from life to death: "And
He breathed into his nostrils the breath of life" (Genesis 2:7).
Similarly, the words *neshimah* (breathing) and *neshamah* (soul
or life) share a common root.[27]

---

25. M. Schreiber, *Responsa Chatam Sofer, Yoreh De'ah*, no. 338.
26. *Mishneh Torah, Hilchot Tumat Met* 1:15.
27. A. Steinberg, *Or Hamizrach*, vol. 36 (1988), pp. 280–289.

The talmudic Sages did not intend to imply that the nostrils determine life, for the nostrils are not an organ upon which human life depends. The teaching of the Sages is that breathing is a sign of life, and that absence of breathing is a sign of death. It is incumbent upon us to identify the organ that controls breathing. The current state of scientific knowledge indicates that it is the brain, and not the heart, that controls breathing.

It follows from the text in *Yoma* and the commentaries thereon that death occurs when breathing totally and irreversibly ceases. The talmudic and post-talmudic sources do not require the cessation of the heartbeat for the determination of the moment of death. Under normal conditions, the time between the cessation of breathing and the cessation of the heartbeat is minimal—a matter of minutes. If there is any possibility of reversing the cessation of respiration and reestablishing independent breathing, one is obligated to attempt to do so by all medical means possible.[28] Under extreme conditions, however, when it is clear that independent breathing can never return because of the irreversible death of the brainstem, the patient can be regarded as dead from the moment that brainstem death is established, even if the patient's heart is still beating.

There is no source in rabbinic literature that states that breathing is dependent upon the brain, just as there is no rabbinic source that states that breathing is dependent upon the heart. According to current scientific knowledge, however, breathing is dependent upon the brain and not the heart. Accordingly, in order to prove that spontaneous breathing—which is the halachic sign of life or death—has irreversibly stopped, it is necessary to prove brainstem death. Halachah requires that the cessation of breathing as the sign of death be final and irreversible. Therefore, Mai-

---

28. S. M. Schwadron, *Responsa Maharsham*, part 6, no. 124.

monides rules that we must wait awhile after the determination of death: "Perhaps the person only fainted."[29] One must confirm that the sign of death is final and irreversible and does not represent a state of transitory unconsciousness. So, too, Rabbi Moshe Isserles, known as Rema, states that we are not sufficiently expert at determining the moment of death of a pregnant woman to allow an immediate Caesarean section to save the life of the fetus.[30] To confirm the irreversibility of the halachic sign of death, the absence of spontaneous breathing, one must convincingly demonstrate the irreversible cessation of the heartbeat or the irreversible cessation of the activity of the brainstem. When either of these situations exists, one can be certain that spontaneous breathing will not resume, and that the person is halachically dead. According to this argument, there is no need for Rabbi Feinstein's innovation that the cessation of breathing due to the destruction of the brainstem is considered equivalent to decapitation.[31] Therefore, this halachic definition of the moment of death—absolute and irreversible cessation of spontaneous respiration—was, and remains, the sole halachic definition. Only the technical means of ascertaining the moment of death have changed.

Recent Rabbinic Responses

The only halachic source that connects breathing to the heart is Rabbi Tzvi ben Yaakov Ashkenazi, knows as Chacham Tzvi.[32] In his responsum he determines two things: (1) *There is no life without the heart* (no one disagrees with this

---

29. *Mishneh Torah, Hilchot Avel* 4:5.

30. Rema's gloss on *Orach Chayim* 330:8: see also E. Y. Waldenberg, *Responsa Tzitz Eliezer*, vol. 10, no. 25:4; Y. Levi, *Ha-Ma'ayan* Tammuz 5731 (1971), pp. 11–18.

31. *Responsa Iggrot Moshe, Yoreh De'ah*, 3:132.

32. *Responsa Chacham Tzvi*, no. 77.

statement);[33] and (2) *The breath comes forth from the heart and is connected to it.* In his words:

> But the breath which issues from the heart through the lung is noticeable as long as the heart is alive. It is very clear that there is breathing only when there is vitality in the heart, from which and for whose needs there is breathing. . . . It is explained that the reason why life is dependent upon the breath of the nostrils is because the hot air from the heart issues forth through the nostrils, and cold air enters through it to cool the heart, and if there is no heart there is no breathing.[34]

Chacham Tzvi cites proofs for this physiological theory from Rabbi Abraham Ibn Ezra, from Rabbi Judah Halevi, author of the *Kuzari*, and from the author of the work *Sha'ar Shamayim*. He concludes: "And all these are agreed, concrete things, with which no one in the world disagrees;" in other words, no one disagrees with this scientific concept as he understands it, and these are all scientific proofs. Although Chacham Tzvi does not cite any halachic source connecting breathing to the heart, he quotes from the Jewish book of mysticism known as the Zohar that it is not possible to live without the heart, but adds that no proof is given there that the heart directly controls a person's breathing. According to current scientific knowledge, the heart obviously pumps blood, and not air.

Chatam Sofer writes that if the reality, as proven by physicians, is different from what has been described to us, even by the *rishonim*, then we must accept the reality:

---

33. But see *Kereiti Upleiti, Yoreh De'ah* 40:104, who states that he conducted lengthy consultations with the physicians of his time and disagrees with Chacham Tzvi on this matter; see also *Darchei Teshuvah* 40:123; see also I. Karelitz, *Chazon Ish, Yoreh De'ah* 40:14, who states that there is no substitute for the heart; without it, one cannot live.

34. Op. cit.

After an investigation from books and authors, and scholars and books of surgery, we cannot deny the reality, which is not as it appears in the commentary of Rashi and the Tosafot and as it was described by the Maharam [Rabbi Meir ben Gedaliah] of Lublin. . . . But after asking forgiveness from our saintly rabbis, their statements were not correct.[35]

He thus adds that matters are in accordance with the expert books of physicians, both Jewish and non-Jewish, and that he had consulted with physicians.[36] Rabbi Abraham, son of Moses Maimonides, writes:

We are not obligated, because of the great stature of the sages of the Talmud and the quality of the perfection of their intellect in the interpretation of the Torah and in its grammar, and the rightness of their statements in the explanation of its rules and details, to accept their arguments and their opinion in all their statements regarding medicine and the science of nature and astronomy, and to believe them as we believe them regarding the interpretation of the Torah, for which they possess the epitome of its wisdom, and to whom it was given over to teach it to the Children of Israel as in the matter regarding which it was written, "According to the law which they shall teach you" [Deuteronomy 17:11] . . . And this is sufficient as a proof and an example that we do not defer to them any more, since we find them making statements on medical matters that have not been verified and that have not been fulfilled in the Talmud: there are many things like this of which they spoke in the chapter *Shemonah Sheratzim* [chapter 14] in Tractate Shabbat, etc., and in other places, things which were investigated by the investigators and which they heard among themselves and upon which they agreed, but

35. *Responsa Chatam Sofer Yoreh De'ah*, no. 338.

36. M. Schreiber, *Chidushei Chatam Sofer* on *Niddah* 18a, entry *Kan*; and *Responsa Chatam Sofer, Yoreh De'ah*, no. 167.

which have not been confirmed by the study of a real physician or by the intellect.[37]

The *poskim* were very particular regarding the honor of the Sages, so that people would not deride words of the Sages that were not scientifically verified according to the understanding of later generations. For example, the *poskim* imposed a ban on using the remedies described in the Talmud because they might not be effective for various reasons.[38] Similarly, they wrote that nature had changed from what it was during the time of the Sages, and that we must accept the reality of science and medicine as it is understood in our time, in halachic as well as nonhalachic matters.[39] One rabbi opines that only when there is a disagreement among the *poskim* is the reality of science effective in enabling us to decide in accordance with one of the conflicting opinions.[40] However, he cites no source for this distinction, thereby casting doubt on the validity of this statement. According to the conception of Chacham Tzvi, breathing is the determining factor of life and death, but respiration is dependent on the flow of air to and from the heart. This concept is not scientifically accurate, since air does not come from the nostrils to the heart. Therefore, since the explanation of Chacham Tzvi of the link between the heart and breathing is contrary to currently accepted scientific facts, and since Chacham Tzvi does not cite support for his position from the talmudic and early post-talmudic literature, we must accept the reality of science as it is known today. Nothing in the halachic literature contra-

---

37. *Al Odot Derashot Hazal* (On the Expositions of the Sages).

38. H. H. Medini, *Sedei Hemed* 200:54.

39. M. Isserles, Rema's gloss on *Even ha-Ezer* 156:4; see also R. Margolioth, *Nefesh Chayah* commentary on *Orach Chayim* 179:61, which provides many examples.

40. S. Vasner, *Assia*, nos. 42–43 (1987), p. 93.

dicts medical–scientific doctrine regarding the brainstem's control over respiration.

Additional Recent Rabbinic Responsa

Chatam Sofer writes that death is defined as follows: "But regarding anyone, after he lies like an inanimate stone, and has no pulse, whose breathing afterwards ceases—it is only on the authority of our holy Torah that we state that he is dead."[41] The sequence, therefore, is total lack of response and movement, followed by cessation of heartbeat, followed by cessation of respiration. This order does not pose a problem for us, for if the heart has irreversibly stopped beating, breathing will immediately cease. However, what would the Halachah be, according to Chatam Sofer, if the patient lies like an inanimate stone, and then breathing ceases, and afterward the heartbeat ceases? Chatam Sofer does not refer to such a case.

Parenthetically, it is possible that the cessation of breathing was followed by the cessation of heartbeat in the case of the son of the Shunammite woman (II Kings 4:18–37) cited by Chatam Sofer. According to several commentators on Maimonides' *Guide of the Perplexed* (1:42), the son of the Shunammite woman was dead, and this was a case of resurrection of the dead, despite the fact that there was still a pulse. During the era of Chatam Sofer, the time difference between brain death and heart death was only a few minutes, and there was no halachic significance in differentiating between them. Today, however, this is not the case. The statement of Chatam Sofer concerning the sequence of events in the occurrence of death does not address the modern-day situation of patients supported by mechanical respirators, in whom total brain death and lack of spontane-

---

41. M. Schreiber, *Responsa Chatam Sofer, Yoreh De'ah*, no. 338.

ous respiration can precede cessation of the heartbeat. Furthermore, the Chatam Sofer himself cites the text in *Yoma* and concludes that the only vital sign is breathing. The Chatam Sofer adds the vital sign of the pulse only in accordance with Maimonides' statement in the *Guide of the Perplexed*. The addition of the pulse by the Chatam Sofer is the addition, not of an essential criterion (because there is no mention of it either in the Talmud or by the *poskim*), but rather of a condition that ensures that the cessation of breathing is final and irreversible.[42] Accordingly, in our time we can replace the vital sign of the pulse with that of function of the brainstem, and arrive at the same halachic goal defined by the Chatam Sofer—a determination that the lack of breathing is final and irreversible. The Chatam Sofer does not cite the Chacham Tzvi in support of his opinion, even though he cites the Chacham Tzvi as a halachic authority in other places,[43] implying that Chatam Sofer did not accept the basic assumptions of Chacham Tzvi.

Of the three conditions mentioned by the Chatam Sofer for the determination of death, only the lack of breathing is an absolute condition, without exception. With regard to the two other criteria—the lack of movement and the lack of a pulse—there are unusual cases in the rabbinic literature[44] in which the Sages established the death of a person who had spastic fluttering of the limbs or who still had a heartbeat, or both. The reason is clear: Only the lack of spontaneous breathing was established by the Torah as a sign of death; the

---

42. M. Schreiber, *Responsa Chatam Sofer, Yoreh De'ah*, no. 338, end of entry *Ve-Nechezi*. See also I. Y. Unterman, *Noam*, no. 13, p. 1, para. 6, which implies that he understood the statement by the Chatam Sofer to mean that the cessation of breathing is the factor that determines death. In our time, however, we must verify that the condition is irreversible.

43. See, for example, M. Schreiber, *Responsa Chatam Sofer, Orach Chayim*, no. 51, entry *Uba-Ze Nire Li*.

44. These cases are listed in the Talmud, *Oholot* 1:6, and in Moses Maimonides' *Mishneh Torah, Hilchot Tumat Met* 1:15.

other two vital signs were added only to verify that breathing had indeed irreversibly ceased. Therefore, in situations in which this verification is possible in another way, these additional signs are not taken into account.

Rabbi Abraham Danzig, author of both *Chochmat Adam* (151:18) and *Matzevet Moshe, Hanhagat Chevra Kadisha veha-Avel* (Customs of the Burial Society and Mourning), states that one should place a feather on the dying person's nose. If the feather does not move, then the person is dead (*Matzevet Moshe*, p. 3). He and other sages did not write that one examines the person's heart or temples for a pulsebeat. Rather, the cessation of breathing is certainly a clear sign of death. The absence of a heartbeat is needed only to confirm that the process is irreversible.

Brain Death and Organ Transplants

Rabbi Moshe Feinstein discusses the question of heart transplants and the determination of death in several responsa, all of which were written before 1980, when the rate of success for heart transplants ranged from poor to fair. In the past few years the rate of success has risen substantially so that the procedure is now medically justifiable. As a result of improvements in surgical techniques, and medical advances such as the use of cyclosporine to prevent rejection of the transplanted organ, heart transplants are now considered standard therapy. In his responsa on heart transplants, Rabbi Feinstein also discusses the determination of death. In the following responsum he strongly opposed heart transplants on the grounds that the surgeon who performs such an operation is liable for murder:

> We have seen that [the surgeons] are not expert in this, for they have erred in all the actions they have done, and also that they are intentionally misleading, for all the people in whom

the doctors have transplanted the heart of others have died within a short time, and it is clear that there existed the possibility of living longer with the heart which was in the patient than with the one transplanted within him; therefore the doctors who did this are complete murderers.[45]

When Rabbi Feinstein wrote that responsum, the success rate for heart transplants was so low that it did not justify the dangers inherent in the operation.

In a second responsum, Rabbi Feinstein wrote:

For we have clarified the matter greatly, and my son-in-law, the rabbi and gaon, our master and teacher Rabbi Moshe David Tendler, has also seen in medical journals that there is no change for the better, even for the person who received a transplant, for we have not seen anyone live a number of years, and even the months that he lives are a life of suffering and pain, and he requires physicians, etc.[46]

This responsum was also written before a significant improvement in the transplant success rate had been realized. Rabbi Feinstein's main argument was based on the potential for a successful surgical outcome at that time. Today, the majority of patients who receive heart transplants live for many years without suffering, returning to a normal life. Indeed, according to Rabbi Tendler, Rabbi Feinstein more recently permitted heart transplantation.[47]

Concerning the determination of death, Rabbi Feinstein ruled that the concept of brain death is not halachically valid, and it is only the permanent and irreversible cessation of breathing that determines death.

---

45. M. Feinstein, *Responsa Iggrot Moshe, Yoreh De'ah* 2:146.

46. Ibid., *Choshen Mishpat* 2:72.

47. See in *Assia*, no 42–43 (1987), p. 71, that the husband of Rabbi Feinstein's granddaughter also attested to this fact. See also p. 192 of this book.

Thus, he wrote:

> But the truth is certainly that the brain's ceasing to function
> is not death, for as long as the person breathes he is alive. It
> is only that the brain's cessation of its activity is the thing
> which will lead to death in that he ceases to breathe. [48]

The standard definition of brain death includes the
cessation of respiration. It is impossible to determine brain
death in someone who still breathes! Therefore, in Rabbi
Feinstein's words, "the cessation of the activity of the brain"
does not mean that this will bring about the cessation of
breathing, but rather that the person no longer breathes. It is
possible that an erroneous definition of brain death was
given to Rabbi Feinstein at the time, or that he considered
only the situation of cerebral death rather than total brain
death. He further wrote in the same responsum: "And it is
possible that since he is still alive, there are drugs in the
world which are known, and others still not known, which
may cause the brain to resume its activity."

Once again the very definition of brain death precludes
the possibility of the brain's resuming its activity; there is no
possibility of such a resumption, because otherwise brain
death would not be established. Brain death means the final
and irreversible death of the brain, including the brainstem,
so that independent breathing can never return, even if the
heart continues to beat normally. If the thrust of Rabbi
Feinstein's statement is that it is possible that a drug or other
treatment may some day be discovered to reverse severe
brain damage, then the same claim could be raised regarding
every definition of death, including the cardiac definition.

In a later responsum devoted to the determination of the
moment of death, Rabbi Feinstein does not mention the

---

48. M. Feinstein, op cit., *Yoreh De'ah* 2:146.

heart among the criteria for the establishment of the moment of death. He writes:

> Rather they [the physicians] should check several times, and if he [the patient] does not breathe, this is the sign of death upon which we rely and do not question; and see *Chatam Sofer, Yoreh De'ah* #338, who explains this at length.[49]

With regard to respirators, Rabbi Feinstein writes that the decisive sign of life is independent breathing (not mechanical respiration). He also describes the cerebral blood flow test for determining the flow of blood to the brain, which is one of the tests for determining brain death even while the heart is still beating. Rabbi Feinstein's discussion is based on the scientific articles written by his son-in-law Rabbi Tendler, in which the latter establishes that brain death is the halachic determinant of death and that the activity of the heart is of no consequence in this matter.[50] (There is a clear link between Rabbi Tendler's scientific articles and Rabbi Feinstein's halachic responsa which cite the former's scientific conclusions in an explicit and detailed fashion.) The reason a blood flow test is needed is to show the total lack of blood flow to the brain, thereby confirming the analogy to decapitation, or "it is as if his head was cut off." There may not even be a need for this test, since whatever is determined by the physician, in accordance with standard medical procedures, as final and irreversible brain death will be accompanied by the irreversible cessation of spontaneous breathing that signifies the moment of death as established by the Sages. At times, there might also be a need for the

---

49. Ibid., 3:132.

50. See the articles by M. Tendler, M.D., in "Annals of the New York Academy of Science," vol. 315 (1978), p. 374; *Journal of the American Medical Association*, vol. 238 (1977), p. 1651; and letters to the editor in *Journal of the American Medical Association*, vol. 240 (1979), p. 109, and vol. 243 (1980), p. 808.

blood flow test or other medical examinations, but in many instances there may be no such need.[51]

Some rabbinic responsa contain factual inaccuracies, which undoubtedly influenced their legal decisions. Take, for example, the following statement: "And in truth, the examination of the nostrils does not indicate the cessation of the activity of the brain, but rather the cessation of the activity of the heart."[52] The absence of air emanating from the nostrils does not indicate the cessation of the activity of the heart, but rather the cessation of the activity of the brain.

Heart Transplantation

The chief halachic problem in heart and other organ transplants is the determination of the moment of death, for in order to improve the potential for success, the heart or other organ must be removed while the donor's heart is still beating. If it can be shown that the donor has permanently ceased to breathe independently, then he is dead. The fact that spontaneous breathing will not resume can be determined by either of two methods: either the permanent and irreversible cessation of the heartbeat, or the permanent and irreversible cessation of the activity of the entire brain, including the brainstem. If the absolute and irreversible lack of independent breathing and brainstem functioning is proven, a continued heartbeat is of no significance and the patient is to be considered dead.

Other halachic problems in organ transplantation include the question of desecrating the body of the dead donor,

---

51. See the article by Rabbi S. Yisraeli in *Assia*, vol. 42–43 (1987), pp. 95–104. In his opinion, there is—in the earlier responsa by Rabbi Feinstein—no contradiction to the basic concept of the centrality of independent breathing as the determining factor of death. By contrast, however, see A. S. Abraham in *Assia*, op. cit., pp. 82–83.

52. E. Y. Waldenberg, *Responsa Tzitz Eliezer*, vol. 10, no. 25:4.

the prohibition of deriving benefit from the dead, and the postponement of burial of the dead. Many rabbinic authorities discuss these questions extensively. The great majority of the *poskim* permit organ transplants if the life of the recipient can thereby be saved. The foregoing considerations are set aside for the overriding consideration of saving a life.

There are also halachic questions relating to the transplant recipient, the most important of which is the following: Will the operation improve the recipient's chances to live compared to no operation? The objective answer today is positive. Most potential heart transplant recipients are so sick that there is no alternative treatment method for them. In fact, most are expected to die within weeks or months without the transplant, but live much longer—often many years—if the surgery is performed. Therefore, the *poskim* should consider a heart transplant operation no different from any other dangerous operation. The later rabbinic authorities, known as *acharonim*, discuss extensively the question of endangering "the life of the hour" in favor of the possibility of "eternal life" (i.e., life for more than twelve months), and rule in favor of granting permission for dangerous but potentially life-saving and life-prolonging surgery or medical treatment. Rabbi Jacob Reischer writes that in a case in which "the expert physicians say that without the operation he [the patient] will not live more than six months, and by means of the operation it is possible that he will live [longer], but the operation is very dangerous and there is a greater probability that he will die quickly," it is permissible to perform the operation in accordance with the majority opinion of the physicians and concurrence of the rabbi.[53]

Rabbi Chayim Ozer Grodzinski, known as Achiezer, ruled similarly, writing that it is necessary to rely upon

---

53. *Responsa Shevut Ya'akov*, part 3, no. 75.

physicians in this matter.[54] These rabbis would obviously permit heart transplants in our time, since the chances of success far outweigh the risks involved.

Other questions have been raised regarding the transplant recipient. For example, Rabbi Eliezer Yehudah Waldenberg, author of *Tzitz Eliezer*, writes that we should question whether this operation, "which was not imagined by our forefathers, can be considered as a medical remedy, and whether [or not] the Torah permits the physician to implement cures in such a manner?"[55] But many major operations performed today and many forms of modern medical treatment were not imagined by our forefathers. Are we, therefore, to refrain from using them to save lives? Rabbi Waldenberg himself does not prohibit open heart surgery.[56]

Rabbi Isaiah Karelitz, known as Chazon Ish, writes:

> The Holy One, blessed be He, created cures even for *terefot* [people or animals with lethal physical defects or illnesses]. . . . Some have been revealed [by God] and forgotten. Everything was arranged and ordered by the Creator at the beginning of the Creation. . . . And it is possible further that it is not only in medicinal drugs and their methods that changes have occurred in our time, but also a change in living bodies. . . . And it is possible that the operations in our time were not effective in the early days. . . . But to give in marriage the [dying person's] wife, they do not give in marriage the wife of whoever has a cure in his time.[57]

In his *Tzitz Eliezer*, Rabbi Waldenberg also writes that the removal of the heart from the patient who is to receive a

---

54. *Responsa Achi'ezer, Yoreh De'ah,* no. 16.
55. Op. cit., 25:5.
56. *Assia,* no. 38 (1984), pp. 10–16.
57. *Chazon Ish, Yoreh De'ah* 5:3.

transplant gives him the halachic status of a *terefah* (nonviable person).[58] Since the transformation of a human being into a *terefah* constitutes an act of murder, it follows that the surgeons who remove the diseased heart prior to the implantation of a new heart have the legal status of murderers. However, this opinion was rejected by Rabbi Shlomo Zalman Auerbach, who argues that the diseased heart that is removed from the patient who is to receive a heart transplant is temporarily replaced by a heart–lung machine.[59] Since the patient lives afterward with his transplanted heart, he was therefore alive all the time and never had the legal status of a dead person. Even Rabbi Waldenberg rules that the question of murder does not apply to open heart surgery.[60] Because there is really no difference in this respect between open heart surgery and a heart transplant, all his arguments regarding open heart surgery are valid for a heart transplant as well.[61] Many operations performed today render a person halachically *terefah*; these include intestinal, brain, or lung operations in which the physicians puncture these organs and their membranes. The Chazon Ish wrote:

> There are other *terefot* in man which we do not know; Nachmanides and other commentators have written that man is cured more [often or easily] than animals . . . and with this we can be at ease with the fact that there are daily instances in which the physicians cut into the intestines, yet the patient recovers and lives a complete and enduring life. Accordingly, the law of testimony regarding *terefot* falls by the wayside in our time.[62]

---

59. Cited in A. S. Abraham, *Nishmat Avraham, Yoreh De'ah* 155:2:2.

60. *Assia*, no. 38 (1984), pp. 10–16.

61. See also R. D. A. Kelig, *Responsa Lev Aryeh* 2:36; and M. Halperin, *Emek Halachah—Assia* (Jerusalem: Schlesinger Institute, 1985), pp. 87–89.

62. Op. cit.

Similarly, Rabbi Moshe Feinstein states that the law of animal *terefot* was given to Moses at Mount Sinai, whereas the rules of *terefot* of human beings change in accordance with the medical expertise and opinion of the time, either because of a change in nature or because of medical progress.[63]

CONCLUSIONS

The halachic definition of death is the total, final, and irreversible cessation of independent breathing. This definition has its source in the Talmud and the *rishonim*, and is based on an explicit verse in the Torah, as expounded in *Yoma* 85a. Two prerequisite conditions for the determination of death are that the person appears to be dead[64] and that confirmation is obtained that the cessation of breathing is irreversible. Temporary cessation of breathing does not constitute death, and the ability of physicians to cause a person to resume independent breathing after a temporary cessation does not constitute revival of the dead. When it is clear beyond any doubt that the person will never be capable of breathing by himself, he is halachically defined as dead. Irreversible cessation of respiration can be verified in one of two ways: either by the irreversible cessation of the heartbeat or by the irreversible cessation of the activity of the entire brain, including the brainstem. In either of these two instances, death is determined in accordance with a precise halachic definition—the final and irreversible cessation of spontaneous breathing.

Under ordinary conditions, death is established by the irreversible cessation of both breathing and heartbeat, for both occur within a short period of time, as was established

---

63. *Choshen Mishpat* 73:4.
64. See *Rashi, Yoma* 85a.

by Maimonides.[65] Furthermore, under ordinary conditions (such as death that occurs at home) it is almost impossible to verify the existence of brain death. However, in the case of a patient on a mechanical respirator, whose independent breathing has already ceased but whose heart may still be beating for hours and days, death can be established on the basis of brain death. Here too, death is determined by the irreversible cessation of independent breathing, but the signs of brain death are the proof of the final and irreversible nature of the cessation of breathing. Brain death can be determined today with accuracy and certainty with the aid of reliable clinical and laboratory tests, after whose administration one must wait a number of hours. The tests should then be repeated to confirm absolutely total brain death. Death is confirmed after a period of time has passed, but it is considered to have actually occurred earlier, at the time of the first tests when the irreversible cessation of breathing was proven. The time of death should be recorded on the death certificate as the time of the first test. This approach is supported by the Talmud (*Pesachim* 91a) and by Maimonides;[66] in both it is stated that a person who removes debris and finds a corpse is retroactively ritually unclean from the time he began removing the debris, despite the fact that he became aware of the corpse only after the removal of the debris.[67]

---

65. *Mishneh Torah, Hilchot Avel* 4:5.

66. M. Maimonides, *Mishneh Torah, Hilchot Korban Pesach* 6:10.

67. See also the statement of Rabbi Auerbach cited in *Nishmat Avraham, Yoreh De'ah* 270:101.

10

MODERN PERSPECTIVES ON HALACHAH AND MEDICINE

Rabbi Mordechai Halperin, M.D.

Halachah (Jewish law) encompasses the entire range of human activity. The thousands of halachot (legal rulings) assembled in the four parts of the code of Jewish law known as *Shulchan Aruch* and in the vast sea of rabbinic literature deal with subjects that touch on all aspects of human life, from the moment of conception to the last breath in this world. Medicine, on the other hand, is traditionally limited in its scope to certain aspects of life. Only recently have technological developments expanded the impact of modern medicine on human life. These developments naturally lead to many new points of contact between the world of Halachah and the world of medicine. The purpose of this chapter is to survey some of those points of contact. The first two sections deal with fundamental matters, and the remaining ones focus on medical–halachic problems in the chronological order of human life, beginning with the inception of life and ending with difficult moral issues relating to death.

CONTRADICTION OR PREJUDICE?

From time to time we are led to question whether it is possible to bridge the gap between modern medicine and Halachah. In this question there lurks a tacit assumption of a contradiction between medicine and Halachah. This prejudicial assumption is based on a misunderstanding of the basic characteristics of medical theory and the essence of Halachah. Halachah is a system composed of law, ethics, and a way of life. Jewish law, the operative element of Halachah, requires the fulfillment of positive precepts, such as paying one's debts on time and donning the phylacteries (*tefillin*); it also involves negative precepts, such as the prohibitions against theft and eating pork and shellfish. Science, on the other hand, is not a moral or legal system. Scientific research (including medical research) is merely a powerful *tool* to investigate the laws of nature, and medical technology is a wonderful tool for saving life and improving its quality. As tools, however, medicine and technology can be put to improper use. An example is the guillotine, which was developed by a French physician in December 1789 for scientific purposes. Nuclear devices, as well as biological and chemical warfare materials, are further examples of potentially improper use of technological or scientific developments. Nonetheless, it is clear that science and technology do *not* contradict human morals, despite the possibility of their misuse. The principle is simple: a tool itself cannot contradict a system of laws and values, but the *use* of a tool can contradict such a system. A word processor does not contradict Jewish ethical or halachic values, although it can be used to write pornography. Similarly, technology and medical science do not contradict the moral values of Halachah, although there are examples of medical practice that stand in opposition to such values. Friction between medicine and Halachah can occur when medical technology is used in opposition to Halachah. Occasionally, a specific social or professional norm may stand in opposition to Jewish law. Such oppositions are not new. In olden times, for example, the concept of absolute slavery was a broadly accepted social norm that was rejected by Jewish law.

HUMAN INTERVENTION IN THE AFFAIRS OF GOD

Medicine poses a fundamental question. In the Torah it appears that health is the divine reward for proper conduct. Suffering and disease are the punishment for sin and transgression:

> If thou wilt diligently hearken to the voice of the Lord thy God, and wilt do that which is right in His sight, and wilt give ear to His commandments and keep all His statutes, I will put none of these diseases upon thee which I have brought upon Egypt: for I am the Lord that heals thee. [Exodus 15:26]

> But if thou wilt not hearken to Me and will not do all these commands . . . I will even appoint over you terror, consumption, and fever, that shall consume the eyes and cause sorrow of heart. [Leviticus 26:14–16]

> And also every sickness, and every plague, that is not written in the book of this Torah, them will the Lord bring upon thee, until thou art destroyed. [Deuteronomy 28:61]

These verses seem to imply that medical treatment constitutes a gross interference in the divine scheme of reward and punishment. Even today, members of certain religions refuse all medical treatment so as not to interfere with "the will of God."

Halachah, however, approves of medical treatment and sometimes considers it mandatory. The basis of the halachic imperative to heal derives from the verse "Cause him to be thoroughly healed" (Exodus 21:19). Our Sages taught "Hence do we have permission to heal" (*Baba Kamma* 85a; *Berachot* 60a), from which it is derived that it is *incumbent* upon us to heal and save life, and that withholding treatment is equivalent to shedding blood.[1]

This unambiguous attitude of the halachah regarding the obligation to heal calls for an explanation. If healing appears to represent an act of opposition to divine will, why should such intervention be permitted?

The homiletical work known as Midrash discusses this matter as follows:

Rabbi Ishmael and Rabbi Akiva were walking in Jerusalem together with another man. A sick person met them and said: "Gentlemen, tell me how I may be healed." They responded: "Take such and such, and you will be healed."

After the sick person departed, the man who was accompanying the Rabbis asked: "Who caused his disease?" They answered: "The Holy One, blessed be He." He asked: "Why do you interfere in a matter which is not yours? The Lord did smite him; why then do you heal him?"

The Rabbis asked him: "What is your occupation?" "I work the land. Here you can see my scythe," he answered. Then the Rabbis asked: "Who created the land upon which you work?" "The Holy One, blessed be He." "Then you are interfering in a matter which is not yours. The Lord created the vineyard; why then do you reap its fruits?"

The farmer responded: "Do you not see the scythe in my hand? If I did not plow and weed and put down fertilizer, nothing would grow on the land."

---

1. J. Karo, *Shulchan Aruch, Yoreh De'ah* 336:1.

"Fool," the Rabbis said, "a tree cannot grow if the land is not prepared. And if the tree grows, it will die unless fertilized and watered. Similarly, the body of man must be tended by the physician with proper medication."[2]

The idea expressed in this midrash is clear. The world was created with a system of natural law. Humans are permitted to use the laws of nature to earn their livelihood and to maintain health. We may engage in farming for our livelihood, and it is appropriate to engage in medical therapy for our health. Human deeds do not detract from divine providence. Similarly, it is not an offense to divine providence to give alms to the poor, for the Lord has many ways of providing for His creatures.[3]

Rabbi Abraham Ibn Ezra had a seemingly maverick opinion on these matters. He distinguished between external injury perpetrated by humans, which one is permitted to treat, and internal disease caused by God, which one may not treat.[4] Although this opinion is not accepted by most authorities, it is important to understand Ibn Ezra's distinction between different kinds of injury. Did he have a philosophical objection to human interference with internal disease caused by God? Or was his opinion based on experience that led him to the conclusion that internal injury is best left untreated so as not to endanger the patient with improper therapy, which was quite common in his day? Rabbi Elijah, the Gaon of Vilna, who was familiar with the standards of medical practice 200 years ago, accepted the second explanation.[5]

---

2. *Midrash Shm'uel 4; Midrash Temurah* 2, quoted in *Sefer ha-Pardes*; cf. C. Kahn's introduction to *Sefer Assia*, vol. 2, ed. A. Steinberg (Jerusalem: Rubin Mass, 1981), p. 5.

3. M. Maimonides, Commentary on the Mishnah, *Pesachim*, at the end of chapter 4.

4. Commentary on Exodus 21:19.

5. M. Weinberger, "Call for Medical Help According to Halachah." In *Emek*

IN VITRO FERTILIZATION AND PARTHENOGENESIS

The number of married couples who are unable to conceive has increased from 15 to 18 percent in the last decade.[6-7] Various therapies are successful in treating fewer than half of these couples. Thus about 10 percent of married couples remain childless.[7]

One of the common causes of female infertility is obstruction of the fallopian tubes, which prevents natural fertilization and progression of the fertilized ovum toward the womb. There are a number of causes for such obstruction, but it generally results from inflammation of the pelvic region (sometimes a complication of induced abortion or pelvic surgery). Techniques for in vitro fertilization, developed during the last ten years, provide means for fertilization *outside the woman's body* and subsequent implantation of the embryo within the woman's uterus. In vitro fertilization requires hormonal induction of ovulation and extraction of ova by means of either a minor surgical procedure (laparoscopy) or insertion of a syringe under ultrasound monitoring. Semen must be collected and prepared for fertilization (capacitation). The actual fertilization takes place in a laboratory. If fertilization is successful, a number of embryos can be implanted in the patient's uterus.[8] This procedure is also effective in certain cases of male infertility, since the in vitro fertilization technique requires fewer sperm cells than does

Halachah—Assia, ed. M. Halperin (Jerusalem: Schlesinger Institute, 1985), pp. 11–34, note 10.

6. S. J. Behrman, "Evaluation of Fertility in the 1980s." In *Progress in Fertility*, 3rd ed., ed. S. J. Behrman (Boston: Little, Brown, 1988), p. 1.

7. E. and B. Lunenfeld, "The Struggle against Infertility," *Madda* (Jerusalem), vol. 25 (1967), pp. 72–75. The statistics cited on p. 75 relate to couples married in 1966. Of these, 12.2 percent remained childless after ten years of marriage.

8. P. V. Dandekar and M .M. Quigley, "Laboratory Setup for Human In Vitro Fertilization," *Fertility and Sterility*, vol. 42 (1984), pp. 1–11.

natural fertilization.[9] The success rate for in vitro fertilization is approximately 20 percent, depending on the exact cause of infertility and other criteria for selecting candidates for the procedure.[10]

Leading rabbinic authorities dealt with the halachic aspects of in vitro fertilization shortly after the procedure was developed. A definite ruling on whether the procedure is permitted by Jewish law is by no means easy to establish. First, one must determine the halachic status of the offspring. Does Jewish law in this case acknowledge a legal relationship between the offspring and its genetic parents? Is the offspring considered legitimate? Does it suffer any halachic disabilities? Does the genetic father fulfill the positive precept "Be fruitful and multiply"?[11]

Answers to these questions are complicated by the fact that in Halachah the relationship between parent and child does not always mirror their *genetic* relationship. For example, the Talmud characterizes converts to Judaism to be "like newborn children" (*Yebamot* 22a). This means that at the moment of conversion, the convert severs his legal relationship with his genetic relatives.[12] This is one example of a genetic relationship that is not acknowledged in Jewish law.

There are also cases in which a halachic relationship exists despite the absence of any genetic relationship. One

---

9. P. L. Matston, "Oligospermic Infertility Treated by In Vitro Fertilization," *Australian and New Zealand Journal of Obstetrics and Gynecology*, vol. 26 (1986), pp. 84–87; D. Martin and R. C. Pan, "Drug Treatment of Oligospermia of Idiopathic Origin: Critical Review," *Annals of Urology* (Paris), vol. 20 (1986), pp. 9–14.

10. P. A. Lancaster, "Obstetric Outcome," *Clinical Obstetrics and Gynecology*, vol. 12 (1985), pp. 847–864.

11. Genesis 1:28; Isaac of Corbeil, *Sefer Mitzvot Katan*, known as *Semak*, Positive Commandment no. 49; M. Maimonides, *Sefer ha-Mitzvot*, Positive Commandment no. 212.

12. M. Maimonides, *Mishneh Torah, Hilchot Issurei Bi'ah* 14:11–15; see also R. E. Mizrachi's commentary on Leviticus 20:17; and Y. Rozanes, *Parshat Derachim, Derech ha-Atarim* 1.

such case is parthenogenesis—the bearing of offspring by the
female without a male genetic contribution. Parthenogenesis
is well documented in the animal world.[13] Is human parthenogenesis possible? Are there human female progeny who
were born without any paternal genetic contribution?[14]
There is no definite answer to these questions, despite
laboratory success in inducing cleavage divisions of a non-
fertilized human ovum.[15] The question is still academic, but
one would have to clarify the position of Jewish law with
respect to the parthenogenetic daughter if such a person is
ever proven to exist. For example, is the mother's husband
considered to be the girl's halachic father, despite the fact that
he contributed no genetic matter? A question such as this
does not have a definite answer, but there are indications that
the girl *would* be recognized as the halachic daughter of the
mother's husband.[16] If so, this is an example of halachic
paternity without genetic relationship.

In the light of these examples, we must seriously
consider the halachic status of "test tube babies." Leading
rabbis are divided on the issue. Rabbi Eliezer Yehudah
Waldenberg[17] is of the opinion that a test tube baby has no
halachic relationship with its genetic parents. He therefore
concludes that the precept "Be fruitful and multiply" is not
fulfilled by the birth of such a child. Moreover, the entire
process of in vitro fertilization, in his view, is halachically
forbidden. Rabbi Ovadiah Yosef (the former Sephardi Chief
Rabbi of Israel) disagrees and permits in vitro fertilization

---

13. U. Mittwoch, "Parthenogenesis (review)," *Journal of Medical Genetics*, vol.
15 (1978), pp. 165–181.

14. In the absence of male genetic material the offspring of parthenogenesis
cannot have a Y chromosome, and therefore such offspring must be female. See
Mittwoch, op. cit., p. 20.

15. Ibid., pp. 176–178; for laboratory experience with parthenogenesis, see pp.
177–178.

16. M. Halperin, "Parthenogenesis in Ashdod?" In *Sefer Assia*, vol. 5, ed. M.
Halperin and Y. Schlesinger (Jerusalem: Rubin Mass, 1986), pp. 179–184.

17. *Responsa Tzitz Eliezer*, cited in *Sefer Assia*, ibid., pp. 89–92.

with the husband's sperm when there is no other available method of bearing children.[18]

Rabbi Avigdor Nebenzahl[19] wrote comments on the opinion of Rabbi Waldenberg, and stated that harmony within the family unit has such great value within the framework of Jewish law[20] that the following should be kept in mind:

> It is proper to remember that if we prohibit in vitro fertilization, we will cause at least one of two things: either the husband will be unable to fulfill the precept "Be fruitful and multiply," leading to ongoing tension and bitterness within the household, or the couple will separate, thereby destroying the household. Perhaps this consideration is insufficient to decide the issue, but in my opinion it seems right to at least mention it.[21]

The point made by Rabbi Nebenzahl has indeed decided the issue for many other rabbis.[22]

It is not the purpose of this chapter to decide matters of Halachah. The interested reader can pursue the matter further by examining halachic sources and consulting competent rabbinic authorities.

It is important to note that recent advances in microscopic surgical technique have made it possible in some cases to open up obstructed fallopian tubes, particularly if the obstruction is related to pelvic inflammation. There are even cases in which the prognosis for surgical treatment exceeds that for in vitro fertilization,[23] and this might influence both

---

18. A. S. Abraham, *Lev Avraham*, 3rd ed., vol. 1. (Jerusalem, 1977), 30: 3; *Nishmat Avraham*, Even ha-Ezer (1987), 1:5 (3).

19. *Sefer Assia*, op. cit., pp. 922–923.

20. *Chullin* 141a (cf. Numbers 5:23).

21. *Op. cit.*

22. O. Yosef, *Responsa Yabbia Omer*, vol. 2, no. 1:12.

23. A. Bremond, et al., "Sterility of Tubal Origin: Microsurgery and Fertiliza-

medical and halachic decisions.

Contemporary halachic literature has considered such subjects as embryo freezing,[24] reduction of embryos in multiple pregnancies (specifically, "thinning" in the case of sextuplets),[25] surrogate motherhood,[26] the halachic status of the offspring of surrogate mothers,[27] and other new techniques for enhancing fertility, such as the Gamete Intrafallopian Transfer (GIFT) procedure.[28]

INDUCED ABORTION AND TAY-SACHS DISEASE

A fetus is biologically alive. Its heart beats from the beginning of the fourth week after conception.[29] Organogenesis, the formation of the body's organs, is complete by the end of

tion In Vitro." *Revue Francaise de Gynecologie et Obstetrique*, vol. 8, (1986), pp. 227–242; K. Luber, et al., "Result of Microsurgical Treatment of Tubal Infertility: Implications for In Vitro Fertilization," *American Journal of Obstetrics and Gynecology*, vol. 154 (1989), pp. 1264–1270.

24. M. Halperin, "Applying the Principles of *Halakhah* to Modern Medicine: In Vitro Fertilization, Frozen Embryos," *Proceedings of the AOJS*, vol. 9 (1987), pp. 197–212; "In Vitro Fertilization. Embryo Transfer and Embryo Freezing," in *Assia*, no. 1 (1988), pp. 25–30.

25. I. Silberstein, "*Dillul Ubbarim,*" *Assia*, no. 45–46 (1989), pp. 1–2; and *Nishmat Avraham, Choshen Mishpat* (1987) 425:1a, cited in the name of Rabbi Shlomo Zalman Auerbach.

26. F. Rosner, "In Vitro Fertilization and Surrogate Motherhood: The Jewish View," *Journal of Religion and Health*, vol. 22 (1983); I. M. Ben Meir, "In Vitro Fertilization: The Legal Relationships of the Embryo and the Surrogate Mother," *Assia*, vol. 11 (1986), pp. 25–40.

27. J.G. Schenkar and M. Halperin, "Jewish Law (*Halakha*) and IVF/ET," *Foundation of In Vitro Fertilization*, ed. C. M. Fredrics et al. (Washington, DC: Hemisphere Publishing Co., 1987), pp. 357–365.

28. S. L. Corcon, et al., "Early Experience with the GIFT Procedure," in *Journal of Reproductive Medicine*, vol. 31 (1986), pp. 219–223.

29. H. Gray, *Anatomy of the Human Body*, 35th ed. (Philadelphia: Lea & Febiger, 1973), p. 151.

the sixth week.[30] Thus, there is no sharply defined point at which the embryo can be said to acquire biological life. The only point in embryonic life that we can identify with any certainty is the moment of fertilization, at which time the embryo becomes a living being from the point of view of the life sciences.[31] It is therefore clear that induced abortion is the ending of a human life. The total dependence of the embryo upon its mother does not constitute any philosophical justification for taking its life, just as the total dependence of a newborn baby on its caretaker does not constitute such justification.[32] The mother's convenience plays no role here.

Among the Noahide laws we find the severe prohibition of abortion (*Sanhedrin* 47b) in the verse: "He who spills the blood of a person within a person, his blood shall surely be spilled" (Genesis 9:6). The Sages taught: "What is a person within a person? It is a fetus. He who destroys a fetus is worthy of the death penalty" (*Sanhedrin* 47b). Nevertheless, the Sages taught that in Jewish law there is no death penalty for abortion.[33] Therefore, within the system of Jewish law one must distinguish between destruction of the fetus, for which there is no death penalty, and destruction of the newborn.[34]

In light of this, there is controversy among contemporary rabbis regarding the severity of the prohibition against abortion in Jewish law. Some hold that abortion is equivalent to murder and that punishment is imposed by God.[35] Other

---

30. *Mishnah, Niddah* 3:7; cf. *Anatomy of the Human Body*, op. cit.

31. Y. Leibowitz, "Medicine and Life Values," *Divre ha-Katedra le Toledot ha-Refu'ah* (Tel Aviv: University of Tel Aviv, 1977), p. 9.

32. Ibid., pp. 9–10.

33. *Mishnah, Niddah* 5:3 (cf. Exodus 21:22–23).

34. Ibid., M. Maimonides, *Mishneh Torah, Hilchot Rotze'ach* 2:6.

35. Rabbi Meir Simchah ha-Kohen of Dvinsk's commentary *Meshech Chochmah* on Exodus 35:2. Additional sources include *Nishmat Avraham, Choshen*

authorities are of the opinion that there is no Torah prohibition against inducing abortion, but only a prohibition
of rabbinic origin.[36] These rabbis hold that the prohibition against inducing abortion does not apply in the face of
severe maternal suffering, in which case one may abort the
fetus.

This controversy touches upon the issue of Tay-Sachs
disease. In this genetic disease, the newborn has a deficiency
of the enzyme hexosaminidase, which leads to the storage of
the lipid called G^{mz} ganglioside, mostly in the central
nervous system. At birth the baby appears entirely normal,
but within several months, as the lipid material begins to
accumulate, the baby's development regresses. Cerebral
degeneration, psychomotor retardation, and further decline
in the baby's condition inevitably lead to death within a few
years. A great deal of suffering is endured by family members when the inevitable result is death of a baby. Tay-Sachs
disease is relatively common among Ashkenazi Jews, occurring in the offspring of one out of every 625 couples.[37]

Amniocentesis, a test of the amniotic fluid during
pregnancy, enables the physician to ascertain whether or not
the fetus is affected by Tay-Sachs disease. There is no doubt
that abortion in the case of a positive diagnosis of Tay-Sachs
disease would alleviate much suffering in the family. The
halachic question is whether it is permitted to take the life of
a living fetus in order to avoid what would otherwise be
severe suffering in the family, primarily on the mother's part.
Rabbi Moshe Feinstein prohibits abortion in such cases. In
his opinion, abortion is equivalent to murder, is therefore
prohibited by the Torah, and is not justified even in cases of

---

Mishpat 425:1a; A. Steinberg, *Sefer Assia*, vol. 1 (Jerusalem: Schlesinger Institute,
1976), pp. 107–124.

36. Ibid.

37. W. E. Nelson, *Textbook of Pediatrics*, 12th ed. (Philadelphia: Saunders,
1983), pp. 478–479.

severe suffering, except when the mother's life is at stake.[38]
Rabbi Waldenberg, on the other hand, permits the abortion
of fetuses suffering from Tay-Sachs disease. In his opinion,
we may rely upon the opinion of those who hold that the
prohibition of abortion is of rabbinic origin and does not
apply in cases of severe suffering.[39]

There are other considerations. In the case of Tay-Sachs
disease, the fetus is in any event doomed to death. Although
the newborn with Tay-Sachs disease has a life expectancy of
more than thirty days, we must still attempt to determine
whether that baby has the halachic status of a *nefel* (a
nonviable newborn considered to be not completely alive).[40]

The consideration of nonviability does not apply to
cases of Down's syndrome (21-trisomy syndrome). Nevertheless, Rabbi Waldenberg found reason to permit abortion
of fetuses diagnosed as suffering from this disorder.[41] Rather
than deciding the issue with a general ruling, Rabbi Waldenberg leaves the ultimate decision to a competent rabbi who
knows the family and can properly evaluate their situation.
The character of the parents and their ability to deal with the
pressures and problems of raising a child affected by Down's
syndrome will weigh heavily in deciding whether or not to
abort. There are families who are able to devote themselves
to raising such a child. The members of such families may
even find that their mutual relationships are strengthened
through the experience of dealing with a Down's syndrome
child. Others may not be able to deal with the pressures. The
halachic decision must therefore take both the medical
situation and the spiritual strength of the parents into

---

38. *Responsa Iggrot Moshe. Choshen Mishpat* 2:69.

39. Op. cit., vol. 13, p. 102, and vol. 14, p. 100.

40. D. A. Kelig, *Responsa Lev Aryeh* 2:32, quoted in *Nishmat Avraham, Choshen Mishpat* 425:1(15); M. Halperin, "Heart Transplants," *Assia*, vol. 11 (1986), pp. 5–29, note 40.

41. *Responsa Tzitz Eliezer*, vol. 14, p. 101.

account. According to Rabbi Waldenberg, therefore, the rabbi most familiar with the family in question must take the final responsibility for the decision.

In a situation in which the mother's life is in danger, there is no controversy. If abortion is the only way to save the mother's life, her life comes first. However, the baby may not be destroyed once its head has been delivered. At that point, the guiding principle is that one life may not be set aside in order to save that of another (*Oholot* 7:6). This principle is discussed in the Talmud[42] and in later rabbinic literature.[43]

Halachic differences between various methods of abortion, and the different periods of pregnancy in relation to its termination, are beyond the scope of this chapter.

PRESERVING LIFE VERSUS FAMILY VALUES

The happy parents had a healthy baby boy. The baby developed and grew into a young man. He chose to study medicine. After years of medical school, internship, and residency, during which he had little time for his wife and children, he was enjoying an opportunity to celebrate the Passover seder with his family. It had been years since he had heard his children ask the "four questions." The family had been looking forward to this night for a long time. The father was ready to relate the story of the Exodus from Egypt and to fulfill the precept "And thou shalt tell thy son."

This was a true family celebration. The house was clean and bright. The special Passover dishes were on the table. Everyone had put on their holiday clothing. All was ready

---

42. *Sanhedrin* 72b; Palestinian Talmud, *Shabbat*, end of chapter 14.

43. *Sanhedrin* 59a, *Tosafot* s.v. *Lekka Midi*; M. Maimonides, *Mishneh Torah, Hilchot Rotze'ach* 1:9. Additional sources include *Sefer ha-Mafteach*, in S. Fraenkel's edition of *Mishneh Torah*, ibid.

for the start of the seder. As his wife was putting the finishing touches on the arrangements, she thought of the traditional question: "How is this night different from all the other nights?" She could not help but think: "On all other nights *Abba* is on call, but on this night *Abba* is at home!"

The seder begins. The telephone rings. The physician, accustomed to receiving emergency calls at all hours, picks up the receiver. He hears the voice of an old man, somewhat frightened: "Doctor, I am sorry to bother you, but my wife insists. It's really not so serious. For three hours I have been feeling a pressure in my chest, and I am sweating a little, despite the cool temperature. Do I have to do anything or can I wait until tomorrow?"

The significance of this conversation is clear. The man was describing what might very well be a heart attack. He should go directly to a hospital emergency room. An ambulance equipped for cardiac intensive care should be ordered at once. The physician would of course advise the patient without unduly worrying him, knowing full well that some 50 percent of all heart attack patients die before medical help reaches them. Perhaps an ambulance will not arrive quickly enough. The physician considers going directly to the patient's home to examine him and treat him on the spot, before the ambulance arrives.

If he decides to go to the patient, he will lose the seder night with his family. The children and his wife will be disappointed. If he drives to the patient's home, he knows that he will have to return by foot, for returning home is not a lifesaving procedure, and therefore he may not drive on Yom Tov. He will not reach home until the early hours of the morning.

In this case, is the physician morally obligated to forgo the seder night with his family? May he rely on the ambulance service to save the patient? Since the ambulance might be delayed, is he halachically obligated to give up his night with the family and go to tend the patient?

In terms of Halachah the answer is simple—saving a life takes precedence over Shabbat and Yom Tov (Jewish holiday): "The zealous in lifesaving are praiseworthy; those who delay treatment to ask whether it is permitted are spillers of blood."[44] Despite all his family's preparations and expectations, despite their frustration and disappointment, the physician father must leave his family and tend to the patient.

A real "lifesaving" procedure takes precedence over Shabbat and Yom Tov, but is a resident physician's routine journey to the hospital included in this category? Does the resident have to avoid desecrating the Sabbath and stay in the hospital during the entire Sabbath and every Sabbath of his hospital residency? Details of the conclusions of Israel's leading rabbinic authorities on this question have been published in the Hebrew journal *Assia*.[45]

EUTHANASIA

In 1962, the following case was brought before a Belgian court: a woman had taken the drug thalidomide during pregnancy. This medication led to the birth of a baby girl with major defects of the arms, legs, and other parts. In desperation, the mother gave her 8-day-old baby sleeping tablets dissolved in milk. The dose proved fatal; the baby died. The mother claimed in her defense that she had committed an act of euthanasia.[46]

"Human vegetables"—terminally ill, comatose pa-

---

44. *Yoma*, chapter 8 (in Babylonian and Palestinian Talmuds); *Shulchan Aruch, Orach Chayim* 328:2.

45. M. Halperin, "Driving In Order to Bring a Resident on Shabbat to Hospital Duty without *T'chum Shabbat*," *Assia*, vol. 11 (1987), pp. 46–51.

46. I. Weinberg, "Euthanasia in Judaism," *Diné Israel*, vol. 7 (1976), pp. 99–127, and especially p. 100.

tients[47]—are not rare in the world of medicine. May we practice euthanasia on such patients?

Professor Yeshayahu Leibowitz offers some incisive remarks on this subject:

If one speaks of mercy killing, one must ask: "Mercy for whom?" A human being has turned into a "vegetable" and has thus become a burden to all around him. It makes no sense to say that we want to be merciful to *the comatose patient* by permitting ourselves to do away with his life, since he is unconscious.

However, there is no doubt that we are merciful to ourselves when we free ourselves of the physical and . . . emotional burdens entailed by the continued care of the comatose patient. Here lies the danger in our decision. If we do away with our fundamental assumption that it is wrong to take human life, if we find cause to justify the taking of human life under certain circumstances, then we know what results are to be expected. It will rapidly become clear to many people that the world is rife with human creatures whose elimination would be an act of mercy. The deception of dealing mercifully with those miserable creatures coincides with the impetus to act mercifully towards oneself. They will eliminate those whose existence they find disturbing. Therefore, I say that even if our sincere emotional response in certain situations of unfortunate human suffering leads us to feel that "death is better than life," we dare not listen to our emotions. The very possibility of our human existence

---

47. Aside from death, there is no concept of "absolute finality" in medical practice. Although rare, there are well-known cases of deeply comatose "vegetating" patients who have regained consciousness despite fatal prognosis. The London *Sunday Times* (December 21, 1986) reported the case of a patient believed to have been "brain dead" who showed signs of life after both his kidneys had been removed for transplantation. See M. Meiri, *Magen Avot* 19, regarding fatal prognoses.

depends upon our insistence on the prohibition of taking human life. Heaven forbid that we adopt the concept of *lebensunwert* [valueless life]. Hitler determined that certain life was "valueless," and he therefore executed 70,000 mental patients and other incurables because their lives were "valueless" and they contributed nothing to society. Hitler thought that whoever freed those miserable creatures from life, and freed society from caring for them, did a favor both to the victim and to society as a whole.[48]

Leibowitz's remarks are philosophical, not halachic: Benefit to society and the value of societal existence require absolute rejection of murder for any reason. Mercy killing is no less than murder.

His distinction between mercy for the patient who has a serious disease and mercy for the relatives of the patient helps to explain an interesting feature in a legislative bill proposed by Israeli Parliament Member M. Cohen-Avidov. In the preamble to his bill, which would obligate physicians to withhold treatment in certain circumstances, he wrote:

Any visitor to an old-age home will be shaken by the sight of those who have lost all function. . . . They are suffering and *their relatives suffer emotionally* because of the condition of their loved ones.[49]

Avidov thus reveals some of the factors that sincerely motivated him to propose this legislation. Mercy for the relatives and visitors plays a significant role in his thinking when he calls for discontinuance of vital treatment in order to hasten death.

Jewish law deals with this painful subject on the basis of

---

48. "Euthanasia," *Korot*, vol. 9 (Jerusalem, 1986), pp. 3–4 and 42–49. Reprinted with permission.

49. Bill 352, submitted to the Knesset on July 7, 1986.

halachic considerations and develops clear guidelines. Murder, the shedding of blood, is one of the severest prohibitions of the Torah. Unlike most other laws of the Torah, which are suspended during life-threatening situations, the prohibition of murder is absolute. One may not take another's life, even to save one's own (*Pesachim* 25b). There is only one exception to this law: in the case of *rodef*—that is, when one individual pursues another with the intent to kill him—it is proper to save the victim. If no other means are available, one may save the victim by killing the pursuer (*Mishnah, Sanhedrin* 8:7).

The value of human life is infinite.[50] Therefore, no consideration, regardless of how reasonable, can lessen the value of life to the extent that killing becomes acceptable. This is so even with respect to mercy killing.

The position of Halachah is unambiguous. Euthanasia is absolutely prohibited.[51] Any action that actively leads to the ending of a human life is defined as murder. On the other hand, a passive influence—the withholding of an artificial device or procedure that is merely prolonging the ill person's suffering—is not defined as murder and is permitted under certain circumstances.[52] The main problem is the precise dividing line between permitted passivity and the kind of "passivity" that is an immediate cause of death. Is withholding food or oxygen considered a passive procedure, or does it cause death? What is the status of an artificial respirator? If one removes an artificial apparatus that is supporting the life of a terminally ill patient, has one passively "removed an impediment" to death, or has one actively killed the patient?

These are hard questions, and they are discussed in

---

50. S. Atlas, quoted in I. Y. Weinberg, *Responsa S'ride Esh* 2:78 (cf. p. 199, section 4); I. Y. Tukatsinski, *Gesher ha-Chayim* 1:2, note 3; I. Jakobovits, *Jewish Medical Ethics* (New York: Bloch, 1978), p. 124.

51. *Nishmat Avraham, Yoreh De'ah* 339:4, s.v. *lachen*.

52. Ibid., note 66.

detail in halachic literature.[53] The leading rabbis of our time are actively involved in elucidating these matters in practice.

SEDATION OF TERMINALLY ILL PATIENTS

Some patients who are suffering from cancer and other potentially terminal diseases may experience great pain. To alleviate that pain, it is sometimes necessary to use increasingly large doses of narcotic substances. These medications may suppress the respiratory center in the brain and might thereby inadvertently shorten the lives of some patients.

In such cases the physician encounters a moral dilemma: On the one hand, he may not shorten the patient's life; on the other hand, the patient is suffering, and the only way to alleviate that suffering is by administering large doses of medication, which may shorten the patient's life.

The Halachah in such situations is unambiguous. It is permissible to alleviate the patient's pain.[54] The decision is easily formulated but difficult to understand. In Jewish law, shortening of life is defined as murder.[55] Euthanasia is also forbidden. Why, then, is a physician permitted to shorten the life of a patient when the intent is to alleviate pain? In the framework of halachic discussions of these principles, some rabbis stress the physician's *intent*. Unlike euthanasia, in which the intent is to kill, administering high doses of narcotic medication for the alleviation of pain is intended to *help* the patient. The shortening of life is merely an undesired side effect.

---

53. For a general survey see A. Steinberg, "Euthanasia." In *Sefer Assia*, vol. 3, ed. A. Steinberg (Jerusalem: Rubin Mass, 1982), pp. 424–457. See also *Nishmat Avraham*, op. cit.; M. Feinstein, in *Moriah*, vol. 13, pp. 52–53.

54. *Nishmat Avraham*, op. cit.

55. A. Nebenzahl, "The Prohibition against Shortening Human Life." In *Sefer Assia*, vol. 5, ed. A. Steinberg (Jerusalem: Schlesinger Institute, 1986), pp. 259–260.

Rabbi Avigdor Nebenzahl rejects this line of reasoning. He points out that in the law of torts (damages) and in the *prohibition* of murder, it is irrelevant whether or not the damage is done by intention. Absence of the intent to kill does not make it permissible to use any procedure that might end with killing. In the conclusion of his discussion he writes:

> I cannot explain Rabbi S. Z. Auerbach's opinion in this matter, unless one were to permit even active killing as a means of alleviating pain. Later I heard him explain that each individual injection does not necessarily shorten life. It is only the cumulative effect of *many* injections which shortens life.[56]

Other explanations have been proposed for this Halachah.[57] Despite the difficulty one may have in understanding the Halachah, it is definitive and is applied in actual cases everywhere.

ORGAN TRANSPLANTS

The human body has many vital organs. These organs, referred to in the Talmud as the "organs upon which life depends,"[58] include the brain, heart, lungs, kidneys,[59] liver,

---

56. "Narcotic Drugs and Critical Patients," *Sefer Assia*, vol. 4, ed. A Steinberg (Jerusalem: Rubin Mass, 1983), pp. 260–262; see also M. Halperin, "Smoking: A Halachic Review," *Emek Halachah—Assia* (1985), pp. 302–311, note 64.

57. *Sefer Assia*, vol. 4 (1983), pp. 263–264; Y. M. Riesel, "Operations with Doubtful Chances of Success," *Emek Halachah—Assia* (1985), p. 1; M. Weinberger, "Intense Suffering with Relation to Medical Decisions," ibid., pp. 53–63.

58. *Temurah 10b–11a*. Cf. *Rashi* and Bezalel Ashkenazi's *Shittah M'kubbetset*.

59. *Mishnah Chullin 3:2*; A. Steinberg, *Chapters in the Pathology of the Talmud* (Jerusalem: Schlesinger Institute, 1975), p. 64; C. Watts and J. R. Cambell,

pancreas, and epidermis. Until recently, functional failure of any one of these organs meant death. However, substitutes have recently been found for some of these organs, and the grave prognosis associated with their loss has largely changed for the better. There are two basic medical solutions for the actual or functional loss or failure of these organs: artificial replacement or organ transplantation.

Examples of artificial replacement include the use of insulin to replace the natural hormonal secretion of the pancreas in patients with diabetes; dialysis to replace the natural functioning of the kidneys in patients suffering from end–stage renal failure; use of a heart–lung machine during open heart surgery while the patient's own heart and lungs do not function; and the implantation of an artificial heart. Examples of organ transplants include transplants of donated kidneys, liver, heart, lung, and pancreas.

From the point of view of Jewish law, medical and technological solutions of the first type (i.e., artificial replacements) are legitimate, permissible, and advisable as long as they indeed increase the patient's life expectancy. In those cases in which only improvement of the quality of life is possible, it is necessary to evaluate the situation very carefully before permitting any surgical procedure that endangers the patient's life. Despite differences of opinion among contemporary rabbis,[60] the patient is entitled to endanger his life by undergoing a therapeutic procedure that is likely to improve his quality of life significantly.

Organ transplants, on the other hand, raise difficult halachic questions. In some cases Jewish law limits the use of human organs. There are fundamental differences between the taking of organs from animal donors, which is permis-

---

"Further Studies on the Effect of Total Nephrectomy in Bovines," *Research in Veterinary Science*, vol. 12 (1971), pp. 234–245.

60. R. S. Braun, *She'arim ha-Metsuyyanim be-Halachah* 190:4; R. J. Emdin, *Mor u-K'tsiah, Orach Chayyim* 328; *Nishmat Avraham, Yoreh De'ah*, 155:2 (2).

sible with almost no restrictions, and the taking of organs from living human donors, which is permissible with certain restrictions intended to protect the life and health of the donor.[61] In addition, it is prohibited to remove an organ from a patient who is on the verge of death.[62] This prohibition calls for a clear definition of the moment of death, since organs may be removed from the donor only after he is deceased. The definition of the moment of death has direct bearing on the permissibility of heart, liver, and other vital organ transplants, as well as on the requisite duration of treatment for comatose patients connected to life-support systems.[63]

Developments in medical technology, together with increased research in medical Halachah in recent years, are leading to practical solutions that were not dreamt of in earlier years. Current halachic discussions of the definition of the moment of death rely on medical technologies that have existed for only a few years. An outstanding rabbi ruled only twenty-one years ago that heart transplants were *double murder*, killing both the donor and the recipient.[64] In those days, the transplant procedure may have actually *shortened* the life expectancy of the recipient. It is therefore not surprising that the initial enthusiasm for the procedure abated—especially in the United States—and human heart transplants were performed less frequently for a fairly long period. In addition, the methods available in those days for establishing the death of the donor were not sophisticated. Some physicians held that reliance on a flat electroencephalogram (EEG) was sufficient to establish the death of the

---

61. *Nishmat Avraham, Yoreh De'ah* 349:3.

62. Ibid., 252:2.

63. See A. Steinberg, "Establishing the Moment of Death for Heart Transplants," *Special Report to the Chief Rabbinate Committee on Heart Transplants* (Jerusalem, 1986).

64. M. Feinstein, *Responsa Iggrot Moshe, Yoreh De'ah* 2:174.

donor. Today, every physician knows that a flat EEG is insufficient to establish death, since it reflects the absence of electrical activity only in the cerebral cortex. This fact does not necessarily indicate death of the entire brain. Therefore, a flat EEG cannot be relied upon as a sign of death of the donor. Many patients who have had flat EEG patterns have subsequently recovered and are alive today.

Contemporary medical technology represents a great improvement over what was available years ago. Today's surgical techniques for organ transplantation are much more refined. Effective new medications are now used for controlling organ rejection.[65] The life expectancy of the recipient of a transplanted heart has increased and is now significantly higher than that of patients who do not receive heart transplants.[66] Methods for establishing death have also been improved by the addition of objective laboratory tests.[67]

These developments called for a reevaluation of the Halachah for heart transplants. Shortly before his death, Rabbi Moshe Feinstein counseled one of his neighbors to undergo a heart transplant.[68] It is therefore clear that heart transplants no longer constitute a case of "double murder," at least in the opinion of Rabbi Feinstein.

In 1986, the Israeli Commission on Transplants, appointed by the Chief Rabbinate, presented its recommendations. The committee included rabbis and rabbinical scholars

65. D. J. Cohen, R. Loertscher, M. F. Rubin, H. L. Tilney, C. B. Carpenter, T. B. Strom, "Cyclosporine A: A New Immunosuppressive Agent for Organ Transplantation," *Annals of Internal Medicine*, vol. 101 (1984), pp. 667–682.

66. Today about 80 percent of all heart transplant patients live more than one year after their surgery, and 70 to 75 percent live more than 2 years (ibid., pp. 673–674).

67. I am referring to the brainstem auditory evoked response (BAER) procedure. See M. Halperin, "Does *Halachah* Permit Heart Transplants?" In *Sefer Assia*, vol. 5 (1986), pp. 55–69, note 55.

68. Rabbi M. D. Tendler in a letter dated July 5, 1986, to the director of Hadassah Medical Center, Jerusalem.

from various sectors of the population, together with two physicians competent in medical Halachah. After protracted discussions the committee wrote the following in its recommendations:

> Since this question touches upon matters of life and death, we feel obligated to establish the position of *halachah* in a clear and definitive way. Relying on the principles of the Talmud [*Yoma* 85] and the decision of the *Chatam Sofer* [*Yoreh De'ah* 338], death is halachically established by the cessation of respiration [see *Iggrot Moshe, Yoreh De'ah* 3].
>
> Therefore, one must establish that respiration has completely and irreversibly stopped. This can be established by proving that the brain, including the brain stem which controls autonomic respiration, is totally destroyed.[69]

The committee recommended accepting, under certain conditions, the recommendations of the Hadassah Medical Center's committee for defining brain death. But they also stipulated a requirement for an additional, objective laboratory test of the brain stem, the brain stem auditory-evoked response known as BAER. This latter test is noninvasive. It involves stimulating the auditory system by sound, and then having a computer decipher the brain waves that originate from the auditory system. If only the "first wave," which originates from the inner ear, can be detected, while other waves that originate from the brain stem cannot, then the ear is functional but the brain stem is dead.[70] In this case, the patient is incapable of autonomic breathing and is therefore halachically dead since Halachah stresses spontaneous breathing as a sign of life. This is the opinion of the Commission on Transplants.

---

69. See "The Decision of the Chief Rabbinate Council," *Assia*, vol. 11 (1987), sections 2–3, pp. 70–81.

70. See H. Somer, "Protocol for the BAER Procedure," *Assia*, ibid., p. 81.

Several leading rabbis declined to participate in the discussions on this issue. Their main reason for refusal was their lack of trust in the physicians and their lack of faith in the ability of the medical establishment to impose obligatory norms.

More than forty years ago, the two then Chief Rabbis of Israel, Rabbi Isaac Halevi Herzog and Rabbi Ben-Zion Uziel, permitted autopsies in spite of prohibitions against desecrating the dead and deriving benefit from the dead *if* the results might immediately save lives. The conditions they established for permitting autopsies have not always been followed, and the law that was subsequently passed has not always been obeyed. There were alleged cases of physicians' signatures added to blank autopsy request forms.[71] Such incidents led to public pressure and a change in the law.[72] In order to deal with problems of physicians not following halachic guidelines, the Chief Rabbinate formulated their decision on heart transplants with a number of administrative restrictions.[73] These restrictions are intended to define the moment of total brain death when the donor's heart continues to beat. Rabbis are divided on the usefulness of these restrictions in the State of Israel. Only time will tell whether the restrictions function as intended.

In addition to life-saving transplants, there are also transplant procedures that can improve the quality of life. Among these are cornea and bone marrow transplants. Also not to be overlooked are "skin transplants" which generally serve as a temporary biological dressing and which can be life-saving. According to Halachah, one is permitted to use

---

71. Report of the State Comptroller, 1969.

72. W. Silberstein and L. Wishlitsky (ed.), *Medical Guide based on Jewish Tradition*, pp. 96–99; *Assia*, vol. 10 (1985), p. 82; *Assia*, vol. 11 (1986), pp. 22–24.

73. See "The Decision of the Chief Rabbinate Council," op. cit., sections 7–9.

the skin of a cadaver in order to save a patient's life.[74] This observation was one factor in the creation of a skin bank in the State of Israel.[75]

The issue of the removal of organs from the deceased for transplantation into living patients is often discussed. Among the most important precepts in this area are the requirement for prompt burial,[76] the prohibition of deriving benefit from a cadaver,[77] and the moral conflict between the personal rights of the deceased and the needs of the living patient. Without consent prior to death no postmortem surgical procedure is permitted. Saving the life of another person is the only reason to violate the body of the deceased without his or her prior consent.[78]

CONCLUSIONS

This chapter has presented some of the many controversial issues in medical Halachah. Other such issues—for example, Halachah in regard to proving paternity by tissue typing,[79] as well as family planning,[80] full disclosure to patients,[81]

---

74. *Nishmat Avraham, Yoreh De'ah* 349:3 (2b), cited in the name of Rabbi Shlomo Zalman Auerbach.

75. S. Israeli, "Skin Transplants from a Cadaver for the Treatment of Burns," *Techumin*, vol. 1., ed. I. Warhaftig (Jerusalem: Zomet, 1980), pp. 237–247.

76. M. Maimonides, *Sefer Hamitzvot*, Positive Commandment no. 231; cf. *Responsa Yabbia Omer*, vol. 3; *Yoreh De'ah* 22.

77. *Shulchan Aruch, Yoreh De'ah* 349:1.

78. *Nishmat Avraham, Yoreh De'ah* 349:2 (2–3).

79. See M. Halperin, C. Brautver, and D. Nelkein, "Establishing Paternity by Tissue Typing (MHC)," *Techumin*, vol. 4 (1983), pp. 431–450.

80. A. Steinberg, "The Jewish Approach to Birth Control." In *Sefer Assia*, vol. 4 (Jerusalem: Rubin Mass, 1983), pp. 139–160; and S. Aviner, "Family Planning and Birth Control," ibid., pp. 167–182.

81. See the articles by S. Glick, Y. Shafran, and A. Avraham in *Assia*, no. 42–43 (1987), pp. 8–15, 16–23, and 24–25 respectively.

geriatrics,[82] and priorities in life-saving—[83]are discussed in detail elsewhere.

I have attempted to present the reader with a sense of the current research in the field of medical Halachah. It is my hope that this chapter will increase the reader's awareness of the values of Torah and ethics in contemporary society.

---

82. S. Y. Cohen, "The Concept of Old Age in Jewish Thought," *Assia*, no. 36 (1984), pp. 13–24.

83. *Sefer Assia*, vol. 3 (Jerusalem: Rubin Mass, 1983), pp. 343–344, 472–473.

INDEX